Praise for

Diagnosed

"Brenda has learned from vast experiences how to make sweet lemonade out of very sour lemons. In this book, she shares her experience in the lemonade production. As a neurologist who specialized in multiple sclerosis, I can state categorically that all people with chronic diseases can learn from Brenda's experiences and her ability to communicate what she has learned over the decades of managing her personal multiple sclerosis journey. Her ability to communicate how to do more than cope but to flourish despite multiple issues is superb! The book does not sugarcoat significant health issues but gives approaches to managing them. It should become an important tool for those with serious health challenges, no matter what their conditions are."

> —Randall T. Schapiro, M.D., FAAN, Clinical Professor of Neurology (retired), University of Minnesota, and founder, The Schapiro Center for Multiple Sclerosis

"Brenda Snow has accomplished something I never thought possible. She has humanized personal tragedy and physical pain and suffering without portraying herself as a victim. There is no whining here about the unfairness of the world. Rather, Brenda uses vivid, vulnerable storytelling to help us understand her journey and then she gives us the tools and strategies she developed to save her own life and eventually help others do the same.

Brenda uses both evocative language and provocative storytelling to keep us engaged. Her self-deprecating but 'in-your-face' writing style underscores the fact that she really needed to share her story. It's clearly cathartic for her and cleansing for those of us who get to immerse ourselves in this book.

Oh, and did I mention that Brenda is funny? Like, really funny. It's a true talent to look at the struggle through a lens of humor. It feels as if the laughter makes the hardship bearable.

Diagnosed is an inspiring story of survival and resilience, but it's so much more than that. It's a blueprint for how to live your best life right now, even in the face of overwhelming hardship. There is no future time when everything will be perfect. The time to start living is today. Just ask Brenda Snow."

> —Charlie Engle, ultramarathon runner, caregiver, and author of *Running Man*

"With compassion and practical guidance, *Diagnosed* will not only help patients and caregivers understand how to advocate for themselves and navigate the complexities of the healthcare system, but also inspire hope and encourage them to embrace a fulfilling life, a life that impacts others, even in the face of adversity. Having known Brenda Snow for eighteen years and witnessed her remarkable expertise firsthand, I can attest to her profound impact on those facing a daunting diagnosis and learning to live in a new normal. Brenda's personal journey and intimate knowledge shine through as she offers invaluable advice and support. You will laugh, cry, and most definitely come to understand that you are not alone."

—Amy Wyatt, epilepsy advocate, writer, and speaker

Diagnosed

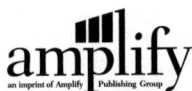

amplify

an imprint of Amplify | **Publishing Group**

www.amplifypublishinggroup.com

Diagnosed: The Essential Guide to Navigating the Patient's Journey

For more information, please contact:
Amplify Publishing, an imprint of Amplify Publishing Group
620 Herndon Parkway, Suite 220
Herndon, VA 20170
info@amplifypublishing.com

Library of Congress Control Number: 2024915851

CPSIA Code: PRV0325B

Second Printing. This Amplify Publishing edition printed in 2025.

ISBN-13: 979-8-89138-195-7

Printed in the United States

*For all those who find themselves on a Journey
they didn't choose. May you discover the tools
and the hope you need to experience a whole,
complete life in spite of illness.*

*And to my girls, Steph and Avery: always know
how much I love you.*

*And to Oliver: this would not have been possible
without you.*

B.S.

BRENDA SNOW

with Greta Myers

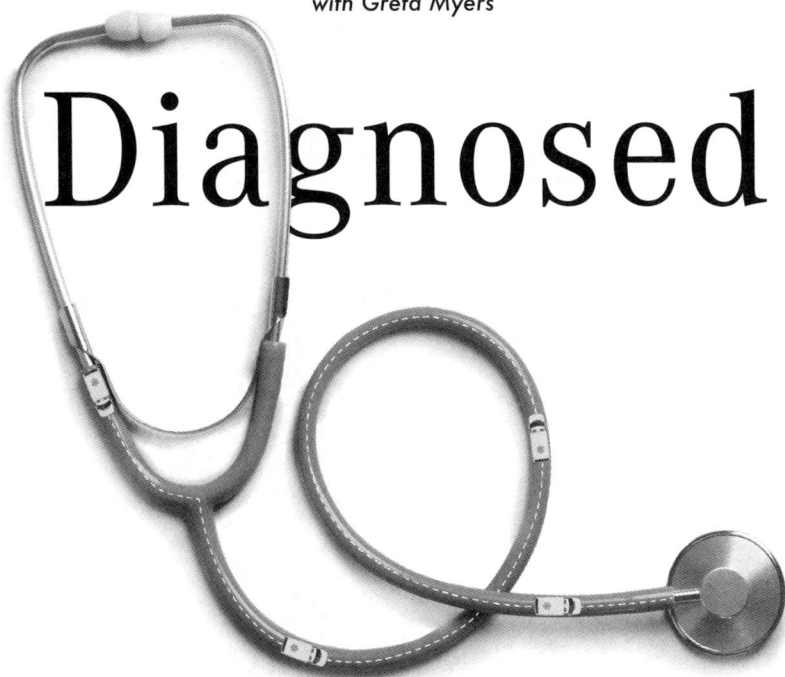

Diagnosed

The **ESSENTIAL GUIDE** *to*
NAVIGATING *the*
PATIENT'S JOURNEY*

with swear words

amplify
an imprint of Amplify Publishing Group

Contents

Author's Note

This book is intended to provide patients with a resource to navigate the turbulent emotional journey that comes when living life with a life-altering disease. However, it is not meant to be a source of medical advice. I am not a healthcare provider, and this book is not intended to provide health counsel or be a tool for diagnosis.

Additionally, my journey with MS has stretched out over thirty years; many of the statistics and data I was working with early after my diagnosis are no longer current. As just one example, my diagnosis—Relapsing-Remitting MS—is now simply known as Relapsing MS.

Diagnostic tools, pharmaceutical options, and terminology have all changed over the years, along with MS patients' experience of the disease: many patients diagnosed today can anticipate a much easier road than I was told to expect in 1993. For the most up-to-date information on MS, please consult the website of the National Multiple Sclerosis Society.

Additionally, this book is not a memoir, although I do share many personal stories. My priority with this book has been to create a helpful guide for people beginning their Patient's Journey. Some parts of my personal story were condensed to maximize the relevance for the reader.

With all that said, please: read, learn, and live. You are not alone.

CHAPTER 1

The Patient's Journey

"You are braver than you believe, stronger than you seem,
and smarter than you think."

— *A.A. Milne*

It's never a good moment when your five-year-old asks, "Mommy, are you going to die?" and you don't know how to answer.

That's tough. That's the moment where you blink back tears and think, *What the hell is happening to me?*

Roughly thirty years ago, all the hopes and dreams I had for my life were upended when my body started to rapidly fail me. At my lowest, I didn't think that I would live long enough to see my daughter reach maturity. And as a single parent, I was devastated to think that she might grow up without her mother's love and guidance.

I'd gone from a vibrant, active, intelligent, engaged person, to someone who couldn't get out of bed. I couldn't control my bladder or my bowels. My left leg didn't work. I had fatigue that was completely unlike anything I'd ever experienced before. I had double vision. And when I brought all these symptoms to various doctors,

I was misdiagnosed, I was trivialized and placated, and one even said I was crazy.

I'd gone from a vibrant, active, intelligent, engaged person, to someone who couldn't get out of bed.

Thirty years later, things look different. As I write these words today, I'm the founder and CEO of Snow Companies, a patient engagement agency that focuses specifically on chronic, rare, and sadly sometimes terminal conditions. We employ 400 people all over the world and work with thousands of Patient Ambassadors who share their stories with other patients to encourage, inform, and inspire them.

Although I'm still living the life of a patient—my particular diagnosis is multiple sclerosis—I've also lived plenty of life beyond the sick bed. My insidious disease somehow brought me into a place of rebuilding and reinvention. It's been hard work, but I've gone from hell, to living with hope, to ultimately experiencing wholeness and beauty in my life.

The best part of my job is that I get to interact with patients. Over the decades I've been in my role, I have been touched and humbled by hundreds of thousands of patients whose stories I've been privileged to hear and learn from. They have taught me about their own Patient Journeys, and we have laughed and cried and swapped tips with one another, all while feeling amazement at what we've been able to overcome.

And: I'm not dead yet! I was able to see my beautiful daughter turn thirty-six this year, and I'm blessed to be a grandmother of an amazing little girl. Over thirty years ago, after getting my diagnosis,

I would never have believed there could be a good life for me on the other side. Yet, here I am. And life is pretty damn good.

After getting my diagnosis, I would never have believed there could be a good life for me on the other side. Yet, here I am. And life is pretty damn good.

UPENDED BY DISEASE

But if you've picked up this book, you might currently relate more to the first part of my story than the second.

A recent diagnosis may have left you feeling absolutely gutted. Fear tends to come first as the *what ifs* flood in. You ask questions like, "What if I'm disabled for the rest of my life? What if my spouse leaves me? What if I can't have kids? What if I can't do my job again? What if I die?" You might feel overwhelmed by everything you need to learn, or all the ways you need to change your lifestyle. Sadness and grief can make you feel helpless—you don't know what to do next. Often, you feel crippling loneliness.

And other times, you might feel angry as hell. You might feel resentful of healthy people who take their health for granted, or feel bitter. You might feel insecure as your body and appearance changes. You're obviously in a lot of pain and that makes you mad, too. You might feel like a prisoner of your disease.

You may already be in the "hell" part of this Journey. Basically, it feels like life is over.

But it's not.

It feels like life is over. *But it's not.*

LIFE IS NOT OVER

After thirty years of living with a chronic illness, and twenty-five years speaking with hundreds of thousands of people managing a chronic or terminal disease, I've become an expert on being a patient. I've seen this Journey enough times that I recognize its stages. Yes: there is a Patient's Journey. Similar to the Grief Cycle, patients tend to journey through a recognizable series of experiences as they cope with their illness and process what it means for their lives. In fact, most caregivers go through the same journey.

I know the ebb and flow. I can plot it out and show you what's coming next. Like the Grief Cycle or even the Hero's Journey, the Patient's Journey has been lived out by enough people that there are familiar landmarks we can follow.

When everything feels out of control, this road map can help you regain your footing. I've disseminated the insights, perspectives, and helpful knowledge—both to patients *and* to care partners—that I know you'll need on this Journey.

This book is for any person who has recently been diagnosed with a life-altering disease—chronic, terminal, or temporarily devastating. My own experience has been with a chronic disease, and that will characterize much of the narrative I share with you. However, there is no less relevance for patients with a terminal or life-altering disease. If anything, these principles hold even greater urgency, because you want to make the most of your finite time.

This book is also for care partners. Many diagnoses impact the caregiver almost as much as the patient. If you're the mom of a little girl with cystic fibrosis, *you're* the one who has to lead both of you through the Patient's Journey. You're dealing with your own grief, pain, and fear. *You* have to be the one advocating for her, because the child can't advocate for herself. The same is true for caregivers of patients in some sort of cognitive decline, or anyone who doesn't have the life skills to manage their own illness. In these cases, caregivers have to navigate the Patient's Journey twice over: for themselves, as they process how the illness of their loved one impacts *their* own life, and for the patient, as caregivers help them navigate their own stages of the journey.

If you're in the role of caregiver, there's plenty in this book for you: the same advice I give to the patient, you also need to adapt for yourself. If you don't take care of yourself in the role of care partner, you will not be able to take care of your loved one, and then it's only a matter of time before all the wheels fall off the cart. Take this advice to heart: you're on this journey, too.

The Patient's Journey is not just for patients; it's also for care partners.

THE PATIENT'S JOURNEY

The Patient's Journey starts with the recognition that something is going horribly wrong with your body and the desperate search for answers. After you finally get a name for what's happening, there's grief: you've gotten diagnosed with some crappy disease that nobody wants, and so you grieve. The journey starts in the lows:

the depressing, painful, angry places. But it doesn't end there. It finds its way to hope, rebuilding, and eventually, impact.

Some people get stuck in certain stages. This journey can be brutal. But I've seen many, many patients get through it quickly and with greater apparent ease than others. They work to let go of their grief, sadness, pain, and anger; they move more rapidly to acceptance, endurance, and rebuilding.

That's why in the chapters to come, after describing each stage, I'll share the strategies that can help you navigate each stage with as much success as possible. You'll speed up the process of getting to the place where you can look back and say, "Damn, I'm doing pretty good."

What does the Journey look like? Here's an abbreviated guide.

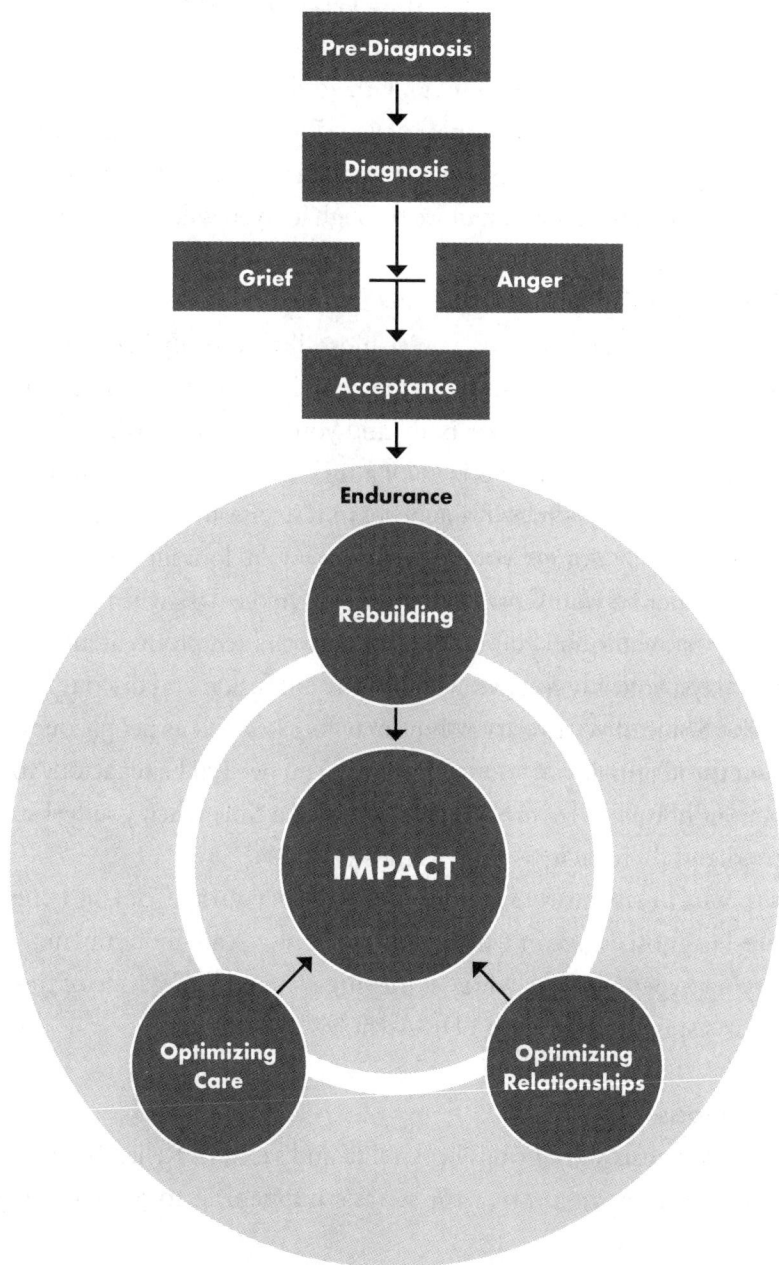

Pre-Diagnosis

Diagnosis

Grief | Anger

Acceptance

Endurance

Rebuilding

IMPACT

Optimizing Care

Optimizing Relationships

PHASE 1: PUTTING OUT THE FIRE

The first half of the Patient's Journey is relatively linear. You can expect to experience each stage in roughly the order it's described. Phase 1 encompasses the early, acute part of your Journey: you're dealing with your body's most debilitating symptoms and putting out the fire. Phase 1 is brutal, but—if you can move through it—you will get *beyond* it.

Pre-Diagnosis

If you're holding this book, you've most likely already had to navigate this first unsettling stage. In the Pre-Diagnosis stage, something weird is happening in your body and you don't know what. Your behavior may be characterized by a mixture of denial and frantic Googling attempts to self-diagnose. Initial trips to the doctor—or doctors—may not get you the answers you're looking for, which can compound your sense of frustration. On the days when you feel your best, you simply don't think about your symptoms at all. On bad days, you may feel overwhelmed by confusion and discouragement. Some of your relationships may feel strained as people question the legitimacy of your symptoms. You need to be tenacious to get out of this stage into the next—but, at a time when you feel so tired and ill, tenacity is hard to muster.

We'll talk more about how to push yourself beyond the Pre-Diagnosis stage in Chapter 2. You'll also read about my mortifying experience in a Macy's dressing room and meet one of this book's starring characters: Dr. Asshole.

Diagnosis

The Diagnosis stage brings both relief and sadness. Relief, because you finally have a *name* for what's happening to your body.

Sadness, because—*what the hell*—you can't believe that this is going to be your life now.

"Why me?" questions tend to rush to the surface in this stage: "What did I do to deserve this? Is this bad karma? Is God punishing me?" You look for someone to blame and often point the finger at yourself. But while that might be normal, it's simply not reality: nobody does anything to deserve a chronic condition.

This stage is also overwhelming. With a diagnosis comes a massive amount of information, and you're usually not up to sifting through it because—duh—you're not feeling well. You're very sick. Many patients experience crushing fatigue and feel generally beaten down. It's not like you have an abundance of energy to go down every informational road and figure out an optimized path forward.

And what makes this all harder is that you're still trying to do all the things you used to do. You're not ready to lean into your care partner yet, or your network of family and friends. You're not turning around and asking people, "Hey, can you help me do this? Can you figure this out for me?" You're still in a place of not wanting to "burden" people. Your entire identity feels threatened—you used to be a healthy person. Now, you're a "sick person." I call this the "identity earthquake."

Complicating all of this is the temptation toward denial that can still characterize this stage. In many ways, you're doing your best to live in a suspended reality. There's still a little bit of disbelief that maybe you made all this up in your head—maybe the doctors got it wrong. Your brain takes a little time to catch up to what your body is trying to tell you. You know you should start processing your diagnosis on a deeper level, but it doesn't yet seem fully real.

We'll unpack all of these complexities and more in Chapter 3. I'll share my own story of finally getting a diagnosis and teach you strategies to shore up your own sense of identity.

Grief

When does it start to seem real? When you're covered and poked and prodded with tubes, blood draws, and more tests. When you're trying to cope with enormous pain. When the medical bills show up on your doorstep. These are ugly, painful moments that confirm: "Yes. I really do have this. This is part of my life now and I can't make it go away."

And then you cry. You feel incredible sadness. You feel grief, depression, even hopelessness.

Grief comes early and it will also come repeatedly. It's more pronounced early in the journey, but you need to prepare for having waves of grief throughout your journey.

This stage is miserable, but it's also really important. It signals you've successfully moved out of the denial that can characterize the first two stages—and it's appropriate. There's a huge loss you're dealing with, and it's okay to mourn.

The only way to move out of this stage is to accept the grief and let it pass through you. And it is important to move *through* it. Some people get stuck here. They play a victim mentality on repeat, and then their mental health suffers, their physical life suffers, and they don't take needed action to get themselves healthier, which means they can end up much worse off with their disease. In order to own your new life and come out on the other side with hope and positivity, you need to find ways to cope with the grief and move toward acceptance.

After giving yourself permission to grieve, choose hope. Even if you still feel shitty, *make choices* that reflect the hopeful belief that things could and can and will get better. Then, align your actions toward that aspiration—I will give you many strategies in Chapter 4 for guidance on how to do that, and I'll acquaint you with my Dad's guiding mantra (which has become one of my own). Take steps that move you in a positive direction. Eventually, your heart will catch up.

Anger

Anger partners closely with grief. In fact, you might experience them simultaneously. A lot of people are angry about what their disease took away from them: their health, their job, their physical appearance, their ability to run around with their kids or make love to their partner. Some of the most mundane tasks that you used to take for granted may now feel completely out of your reach—and that might make you fucking pissed! Adding insult to injury, you may get irritating or infuriating responses from other people: a lack of support from your boss, or stupid comments from your neighbor, or a patronizing attitude from doctors who treat you like an idiot. There's a lot to be angry about!

But the silver lining of Anger is that there's some energy there. If you use anger to fuel your hope and choices, it can drive you to get out of bed every day and work toward healing. Anger was a big driver for me in moving forward. It motivated me to seek out better answers. It motivated me to tell my story to other people as a cautionary tale: "Don't let this happen to you." It motivated me to seek out other healthcare professionals who would listen to me and take me seriously.

However, this is also a place where people can get stuck. Some people stay bitter and cynical: angry at the world, angry at their doctors, angry at their condition, angry at themselves. But it's a dangerous place to get stuck, because that attitude can prevent you from taking necessary action toward healing. In Chapter 5, we'll discuss much more about the Anger stage and I'll give you concrete steps to help you get unstuck. You'll also hear about a kindergarten showdown and the inglorious time I cussed out the Man in the Yellow Hat.

Ironically, people stay in the Anger stage because it gives you the feeling that you're somehow still maintaining some control. But actually, you get far more control when you move into Acceptance.

Acceptance

Acceptance is hard. I don't want to sound like Pollyanna here. Accepting your illness, to some extent, feels like letting it win.

But at some point, even if you don't *want* to accept the conditions of your illness, you just get too tired to fight it anymore. You get so sick of the parade of negative emotions—the anger, the disbelief, the grief—that eventually, a light bulb goes off. You think, "Maybe it's easier to do it another way."

There's not much you can control in the early phases of chronic and terminal illnesses, but one thing you *can* control: the glasses you put on to perceive your reality and determine the way you show up. You can choose how you see the world.

The minute you stop blaming other people and conclude, "Actually, *I* control part of this," that's the moment you allow yourself to become an empowered, informed, participatory patient. All the energy you had been directing toward anger can now be directed toward doing your therapy exercises or optimizing your care plan. You repurpose that negative energy in a positive direction to *engage*.

When you accept your illness and recognize that some things are beyond your control, you *open* yourself to more effectively control the things that are within your power. In Chapter 6, I'm going to help you hold the hand of this disease and learn how to hate it less, so you can love yourself more. You'll hear about the list of anti-pity-party rules I posted outside my hospital room and understand why Acceptance is such a key element of learning to embrace life again.

By crossing this crucial threshold of Acceptance, you enable yourself to move into the second half of your Patient's Journey and put Phase 1 behind you.

PHASE 2: THE REST OF YOUR LIFE

Phase 2 is not linear, because you will engage in every one of these latter stages for the rest of your life. They may occur simultaneously or in a different order. However, you can trust they *will* follow Phase 1. You won't have the energy you need for any of these latter stages until you turn the corner of Acceptance.

You can also trust that there will be a current pulling you along during this second phase. The skills, tools, and strategies you develop during Endurance, Optimize Your Relationships, and Optimize Your Care will all culminate in Rebuilding and then Impact. And if your journey is anything like the thousands of Patient's Journeys we hear about from our Patient Ambassadors, you will get to a stronger and more beautiful place on the other side of this journey than the life you had before it began.

Endurance

Endurance will characterize much of your Patient's Journey: Endurance during setbacks. Endurance through flare-ups. Endurance as you deal with new, weird symptoms. You will need to *endure* your illness on a regular basis, because just when you think you've got the nut cracked, you'll realize there's some new shit you've got to figure out. Of all the Patient's Journey stages, this is the one that lasts the longest.

Endurance isn't a passive state—think of it as active *retooling*. There are three big areas where you need to build endurance so that you can live your best life for the long haul.

- **First:** Your own self-care. You need to learn your new body and figure out what you need to do to optimize your health. What triggers your flare-ups? How much sleep do you need? When is your best time of day to do tasks that require a higher level of energy?
- **Second:** You need systems and processes in place to build a lifestyle that is more conducive to your new limits. One of the biggest steps you can take in this area is good boundary setting. You need to learn how to say no to people, let them know you can or can't do certain things, and give feedback to correct their wrong assumptions. You also need to have conversations with your family members around division of labor to rebalance chores, tasks, and calendar appointments.
- **Third:** You need to think about your people—because they have a lot to endure as well. It's a hard reality to face that while you *don't* have a choice about living

with illness, your loved ones do. They can opt out—and unfortunately, I've seen many relationships and marriages end because the care partner just couldn't endure. If you want your relationship to make it, then both care partners and patients have a lot to do in this area: communication is huge. And the care partner's self-care is also critical—which the patient would be wise to encourage and support. By taking care of one another, you help give yourself endurance to craft your best shared life possible.

Expect that you will need to continue developing your endurance skills in all three of these categories for the rest of your life. Continue to hone your practices of self-care, your processes for a sustainable lifestyle, and the ways you prioritize your loved ones' self-care. Endure new setbacks with resilience, continue to choose positivity (even if it's with grim resignation), and retool to keep moving forward. We'll discuss these strategies much more in Chapter 7 when we focus on Endurance.

Optimize Your Relationships

The Patient's Journey instigates profound changes in patients, care partners, and everyone touched by the disease; it also causes relationships to evolve. Everyone must learn new roles and new ways of engaging with one another: your partner is now also your caregiver; your best friend is now your chief researcher; your kid becomes your wheelchair docent. These evolutions can be challenging. Illness and disease can be incredibly hard on connection—but they can also open you to opportunities to connect with your loved ones on a *deeper* level.

You're also going to be forming relationships with a lot of new people, starting with your team of health practitioners. You've got to line up the right doctors, specialists, therapists, and so on. Managing all of those new relationships requires energy; in some ways, all of your appointments and new relationships can feel like its own full-time job. And in addition to all of those "required" people, you might find yourself with a new "family": a host of new acquaintances that also have your disease. You may need a legal team in place to help you navigate all the insurance work, especially if you lost your job. You might lose some friends—the ones who just *don't* get it—and gain others: the surprising ones who do.

In other words, you'll have a lot of different relationships that the average person doesn't have to manage. It's ironic that in a time when you're feeling sick, exhausted, in pain, and all the rest, you have more on your plate than you've ever had before. You have *less* energy for relationship management and *more* relationships to manage.

That's why communication becomes really important in this stage. Learn to communicate when your energy is spent, or when you need to clarify that you have enough bandwidth to do exactly *one* thing, whatever it may be. Trying to manage all your relationships without those guardrails in place will take you back to feeling completely overwhelmed and full of fear. But strong communication will do a lot to keep your relationships healthy. The strategies you hone in this stage will continue to help you navigate relationships throughout the different seasons of your illness and life. We'll examine these strategies in Chapter 8 and I'll share how some of my own relationships had to evolve.

Optimize Your Care

Once you've gotten beyond the initial chaos of the acute Phase 1, you get to a place where you can more clearly evaluate your needs and continuously optimize your long-term options. This stage is characterized by learning and self-advocacy, in the interest of optimizing your healthcare and well-being.

What sorts of things are you learning about? You might decide you want to seek out a different medication, or therapy, or doctor. You might learn about alternative treatment modalities. Perhaps you seek out advocacy organizations that can help you navigate the social security fine print, or provide pro bono legal help. You're hunting down the right people to help support you, like the best specialists, or the right marriage counselor, or the friend who's willing to call your healthcare team every morning to see if you can get an appointment any earlier than next month.

While optimizing your care, you will become an expert in areas you probably knew nothing about before getting diagnosed. As you learn more about the best therapeutics, or clinical trials, or disability benefits—you will become a more empowered patient. You will begin to take a more active role in the plan for managing your disease and your life. That's a key element of the Optimize Your Care phase: forming the plan, and then refining the plan.

You'll need to keep tweaking, retooling, and revisiting the plan to architect your Best-Case Scenario as you move through different seasons of life and as your disease potentially changes or new treatment protocols become available. In the Optimize Your Care stage, you're asking with real objectivity, "What's the best plan for my life, right now?"

This stage—like the Endurance and Optimize Your Relation-ships stages—is not linear. You will revisit and refine it often. There are multiple layers of Optimize Your Care, and to some extent, you will be revisiting this stage for as long as you live.

I'll be candid: there's a lot of shit you need to learn about deal-ing with this illness, and Chapter 9 will school you. I'll also share about my Hail Mary attempt to get myself out of debt. (Which ultimately scored!)

Rebuilding

Up to this point, your disease may have cast a pall over your life that makes things feel scary and serious nearly all the time. But there's tremendous stabilizing that occurs in the Endurance, Opti-mize Your Relationships, and Optimize Your Care stages. That means you can finally start to relax a little in the Rebuilding stage—and I recommend you lean into that with gusto.

Rebuilding is all about architecting fun and normalcy back into your life. Life is too short to be serious all the time, and that's a truth you now know with greater sureness than you ever have before. So, plan ways to inject fun and joy into your pre-cious time. Plan vacations. Surround yourself with people who "get it," who can make you laugh. Lean into the deep truths you've discovered during this journey as you've gathered knowl-edge about what's truly meaningful and important. You may feel freedom to reinvent yourself or your pursuits during this stage because of the increased clarity you now have about what's really relevant to you. Go for it! If you're going to expend precious time, energy, and resources doing anything, you want it to *mat-ter*. You want to feel real purpose in it. You don't want to waste time doing stuff that doesn't "count" anymore. You want to enjoy yourself!

Every human being's time on this planet is finite, but on this side of the Patient's Journey, you *know it*. So, you choose laughter. You choose purpose. You choose fun. You choose to make memorable moments. You recognize that you have special talents and skills, and this is your opportunity—*right now*—to go out and build something meaningful. So, as you rebuild, you are choosing, selecting, picking the people and pastimes that have utmost importance to you. In this stage, life begins to take on a feeling of richness beyond measure.

In Chapter 10, you'll learn how to cultivate this richness in your life. I'll also introduce you to my mother, the Queen of Fun, as we all take a lesson from her playbook and consider the merits of Elvis impersonators at a funeral.

Impact

And now, patients begin to ask, "What am I going to do with it? How am I going to give back and leave the world a better place?" That's when you arrive at the Impact stage of your Patient's Journey.

As a patient, you've been freshly and brutally reminded that we're all going to die one day. That universal truth now has personal immediacy to you because death seems like it might be coming a hell of a lot quicker. Nobody wants to think about that—at all. But there's a gift when you make peace with that possibility: you begin *enjoying* your time here more, the sweetness of it. And you develop a strong desire to make a positive impact in any way you can.

I've stood on a stage in front of thousands of people, sharing my story. Every time I give a talk, I have one goal: if I touch one person's heart or help a single person, that's a win for me. And as I met with patients, one after another, they all said the same thing: "If I can help or make an imprint on just one other person, sharing my experience will be worth it." I've heard that more times than I can count.

It is *powerful* when a person shares what they've gone through—the change, the heartache, the fear, the pain—and then stands up with vulnerability in front of their cohorts and say, "This happened to me, and I want to share it with you." If you pass on one nugget that made *your* journey easier, you have the power to make someone else's journey a little smoother. That's why I've built a company that provides a platform for patients to connect with other patients and share their stories. And it's why, as I delve more fully into each of these stages in the chapters to come, I share my own story with you.

Illness is brutal, but when you start finding ways to give back to others, that impact makes it all easier to bear. It makes it better. It makes it more real. You realize that helping others actually helps *you*.

Impact is our focus in Chapter 11, where you'll learn much more about embracing the avenues of purpose this disease has opened for you. I'll share more about my own experience as founder and CEO of Snow Companies, and my hope is you will find your voice and share your story. You'll end this book feeling inspired and encouraged!

WHAT TO EXPECT

I've listed the stages of the Patient's Journey in the order they most often arrive, but don't expect this to be a tidy experience. You've experienced enough by now to know that very little of the Patient's Journey is tidy. Use this book as it is most practical for you. For instance, if you're dealing with relational struggles, feel free to jump ahead to Chapter 8, Optimize Your Relationships. We'll get through this Journey together. You'll find in this book an honest, first-person perspective of how to navigate the Patient's Journey, not only for you as the patient, but also for your family, loved ones, and friends. I've chosen to share quite a bit of my own story, along with stories from other patients I know, because stories remind us that we're not alone.

I've chosen to share quite a bit of my own story, along with stories from other patients I know, because stories remind us that we're not alone.

I've tried to make it approachable. (That's my nice way of saying I swear a lot.) Lots of parts are funny, because hell, we're dealing with enough serious stuff already. If you're feeling shitty when reading this book, you'll be glad there are a few funny moments in here.

You will find helpful, relevant knowledge that you can easily implement into your own unique situation, whatever that may be. You won't find specific medical advice, because I am not a doctor, nor am I a healthcare professional. I can't treat you, give you specific information about how to get your drugs covered, or explain how to access the most cutting-edge therapeutics—although, I will point you in the right direction.

Think of this book as a companion and as a friend. There's plenty of scary stuff you're working through outside of this book, so I'm not going to pile it on here. This book will make you feel better.

Trust in the wisdom in this book—it reflects the hard-won insight of hundreds of thousands of patients who have already walked this road. Try to implement the strategies I give you—they will help you navigate this Patient's Journey faster and with greater ease. They will get you unstuck from those wallowing swamps that can cause your Journey to get mired in the muck.

And do not give up. This book will inspire you to dig deep, to overcome, and to realize that you are worth it. There's still an amazing life in front of you, for however long it lasts. You should not believe the negative narrative in your head that says you aren't worth fighting for. My hope for everyone reading this book is that you love yourself enough to fucking try.

This book will inspire you to dig deep, to overcome, and to realize that you are worth it. There's still an amazing life in front of you, for however long it lasts.

WHY LISTEN TO ME?

I think you should listen to me because, first of all, I love it when people listen to me. To say I have control issues is an understatement! I want you to listen and let me help control your life so that *it becomes better.*

I have reasons beyond being a control freak. I've walked this road. I've lived with multiple sclerosis for most of my adult life, from the shittiest moments to the best moments. And amazingly—this many years into being a patient—life has turned out to be a beautiful tapestry. Woven into that picture are the shining threads of all the patients I've worked with, within my sphere of influence. I've been blessed to hear countless stories from patients across the globe. Do you know something amazing? Illness transcends skin tone, language, socioeconomic backgrounds, and cultural barriers. As awful as it is, it is a unifier of people. I've been able to hold the hands of people whose language I don't understand, but we each comprehend the impact of illness. Beyond words, we're able to exchange empathy, help, and support. And through my business, I've been exposed to some of the most incredible thought leaders in different diseases: researchers, drug developers, leading advocacy organizations, and so on. I've been privileged to touch many parts of the health ecosystem, experiencing them both as a patient and as a patient advocate.

Through all these different touch points, I've been able to glean quite a bit of knowledge. As part of the legacy I want to leave behind, I want to pass that on to you. I want to make your *own* Journey just a little bit easier. Everyone deserves to have a whole, happy life.

A GLIMPSE OF YOUR FUTURE

You will not believe me now if you're just starting this Journey, but in the weeks, months, and years to come, things will come to look very different. You are joining an exclusive club of brave people who have gone on to experience tremendous meaning and impact in spite of—and often, *because* of—their diagnoses. In their company, you will come to know that you can still have a profoundly beautiful existence for as long as you're still here.

This Journey will remind you of important things: what is good, true, and beautiful about you; what you value most; the fact that you *can* choose hope and optimism, so that you can make positive choices that improve your health. And there are other gifts: your most precious relationships can be strengthened and deepened; they can be taken to new levels of beauty. With the dramatic change in perspective brought on by this hard, hard circumstance, you will discover greater patience, tenderness, empathy, and levity in you. You'll stop sweating the small stuff. You'll feel more gratitude for every moment. You will recognize the value that you have to contribute and the ways you can make an impact on the world.

And you will be empowered with new skills: the skills to pursue happiness, joy, and positivity in your life; the skills to self-advocate so that you can push back against asshole doctors, or roadblocks in the healthcare system, or discrimination for being a patient. You will be an empowered information seeker, so that you know how to get the necessary knowledge to take care of your body. You'll identify necessary boundaries and daily practices that will help you optimize your energy where it counts the most. You will live with a mixture of transparent vulnerability and aggressive self-advocacy. You're a badass patient; an open book; a loving friend, partner, and family member.

And here is what you are *not*: you are not your disease. That is something you will come to know as deeply true. You are a whole person, who *happens* to live with disease as one of your many traits.

These gifts don't happen by accident. You need to do the work and stay positive. But as you do, life will become rich with meaning—it might even be better than before your disease. And when you look around and realize life has become everything I just described, you will look back and say, "Damn. Brenda was right!"

This doesn't happen by accident. You need to do the work and stay positive. As you do, life will become rich with meaning.

I know this to be true because I never, ever, ever thought my life would be worth anything or be any good when I was at my lowest, shortly after my diagnosis. That first year was a full year of hell. Even looking back on it now, I feel rocked to think of what I had to get through.

But I kept moving. I kept walking—or rather, rolling in my wheelchair—along my Patient's Journey. I discovered a life of profound meaning, joy, and impact on the other side and the vast majority of other patients I've talked to have said the same thing. They have gone before you to blaze this trail and they possess tremendous wisdom to share with you, if you're open to hearing it. I may not have all the answers, but I think I have a lot of the answers. And I can assure you that every word in this book comes with the biggest heartfelt virtual hug for you as you start learning more.

I'm eager for you to move beyond the agonizing place you may be right now, and I'm so *excited* for you to experience hope and wholeness. I want you to be able to look back and have the perspective I promise will eventually come, when you can say, "I'm on the other side. And I'm better for having gone through it!" That's my hope and my goal for you: that you would get to a much better place at the end of this Journey—one where you can look at your life in awe, and recognize that it is rich, and full, and whole.

Keep an open mind. Remember you are not alone. Buckle up; let's fucking do this. I believe in you.

PART 1

Putting Out
the Fire

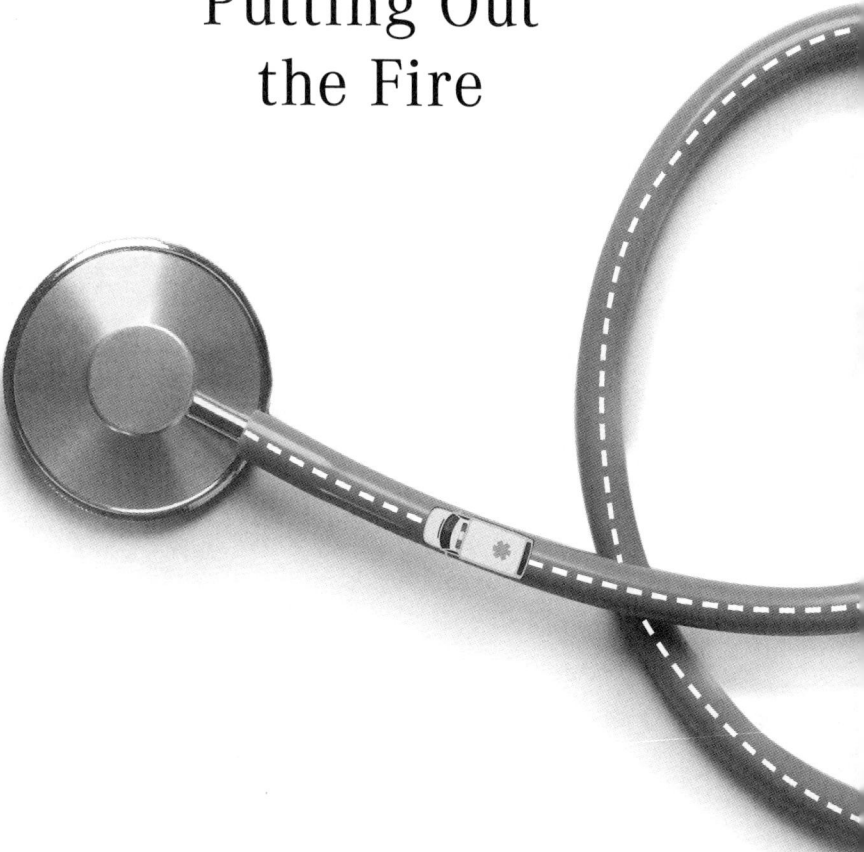

CHAPTER 2

Pre-Diagnosis

IF YOU'RE READING THIS, YOU'RE ALREADY IN IT

"Fear of the unknown is the greatest fear of all."

— *Yvon Chouinard*

It may have started with just one strange symptom—one you could initially laugh off. Then it got worse. You may have started Googling your symptoms. Maybe you met with your Primary Care Physician and left disappointed after realizing they weren't going to give you an easy answer. The symptoms got worse. You felt increasingly desperate to know what the hell was going on with your body.

I see your pain. I know it. I've *lived* it.

You are entering a big fucking trial.

You have begun a journey I'm deeply familiar with: the Patient's Journey. In bearing witness to the many stories other patients shared with me over the last three decades, I've seen patterns emerge. It's a journey that starts from where you find yourself right now, and takes you to where you'll be able to rebuild your life and make a difference in the lives of others.

But I haven't just witnessed the Patient's Journey. I've had to walk the journey firsthand—starting over thirty years ago with the confusing and terrifying symptoms that first alerted me that something in my body was going very, very wrong.

OMINOUS SYMPTOMS AND AN ASSHOLE

September 1993. Desktop computers were a new thing. I was sitting at my desk, responding to emails for my job. Suddenly, the computer split in two. I saw duplicate computers, side by side.

I blinked. The two computers stayed. I reached out my arm to touch them, to see if they were both real. Suddenly I had two right arms. I closed my eyes again and shook my head. I opened my eyes. The two computers had merged back into one.

Slightly rattled, I turned to my coworker and guffawed. "These desktops are not going to be successful in the workplace if they make your eyes go bad!" She looked back at me, confused, then turned back to her own computer.

It happened again and again. I would be looking at something and, all of a sudden, see the world in duplicate. Sometimes, I would be reading text and then holes would appear in the middle of the words—dark places where I couldn't see, like Swiss cheese.

First, I went to an optometrist to get my eyes checked. "There's nothing wrong with your eyes," they told me. "You're too young for readers." I was told it was eye fatigue. "Blame the computer, I guess."

The exhaustion came next. I'm a high energy person—for my entire life, I had been able to maintain strong energy, even when I wasn't getting a lot of sleep. But I was having *overwhelming* fatigue.

I found myself wishing for the days in elementary school when I could go to the nurse's office and take a nap.

Along with the transient vision and this creeping fatigue, I started to notice that my left foot constantly felt cold. Eventually, it stopped feeling cold and just went numb. After several weeks of that, it occurred to me that my foot wasn't working as normal. This felt strange to me. "I used to move my foot," I remarked to my dad one night.

"You don't move your foot anymore?" he asked.

"My foot feels so weird. I can't feel it. And the numbness is starting to come up my leg."

Dad looked concerned. "I think you should see a doctor," he said.

I made an appointment, and in the meantime, I did my best to continue life normally. One day, I had to go to Macy's with my five-year-old daughter, Stephanie. We were in the dressing room when Stephanie said, "Mommy, are you going potty?" I looked down. There was a puddle of urine at my feet. With no sensation in my left leg, I hadn't even noticed something running down my legs. I just stared at the floor in disbelief. My face burned. I felt total humiliation.

A lady outside the dressing room called, "Do you need help?"

I thought, *What the hell am I going to do?! How am I going to get out of this dressing room with my soiled clothing and urine everywhere … ?* I felt a personal responsibility to the store to clean it all up—but I had nothing to clean it with. I was too embarrassed to call out to the woman, "Excuse me, I've just peed all over this dressing room."

I told Stephanie to come with me, dragged my leg out the room, and just … left.

I was getting more and more freaked out. Before the appointment, things continued to escalate. My leg got worse—like the entire limb had just fallen asleep. It wasn't the tingly feeling though, it was the "completely dead limb" feeling. My gait changed. I couldn't walk normally anymore. I dragged my left leg when I walked into the doctor's office.

"It could be sleep deprivation," my primary care physician suggested. "You're a single mom. You're trying to raise a kid and be a career woman. You might just need more rest." He nodded. "Sleep deprivation does incredible things." Then he had another inspiration. "Or it could be a pinched nerve? You're sitting at a desk eight hours a day, when you used to be up and around. Maybe that's it."

I thought about that. "I'll get more rest," I concluded. He nodded. I went home, resolving to go to bed earlier.

But the symptoms got worse. One day, I had the sensation that someone sawed me in half at the waist and then poured concrete down my left leg. It felt like this incredibly heavy appendage that I had to just drag around.

I made another appointment and mentioned the escalating symptoms, including my issues with urination. The doctor had an easy answer for that one: "That's just from your pregnancy. You're only a few years out. That can happen to women after they have a baby."

"But I had a C-section," I protested.

He waved that off. "It's a postpartum thing."

In my gut, I believed it was *not* just a postpartum thing, and by now, I had started to panic. A family friend had mentioned MS, so I made an appointment with a neurologist, once again dragging my leg behind me into our first appointment. I told him, "I can't feel my leg. It won't move. I'm exhausted. I have double vision. I can't control my bladder. What is going on with me?!"

He studied me, his head cocked to the side. "I think it's migraine headaches," he said.

I took a slow, ragged breath. I responded, "But on my intake form, I didn't check the headache box. I do not have a headache."

He said, "You know, migraines can do lots of things." He wrote me a prescription for the newest FDA-approved drug for migraines. "Go take this."

I stared at the prescription. I knew I wasn't going to go fill it. I wanted to say, "I don't have a headache, but *you* are giving me a fucking headache." I didn't say that, though. I meekly thanked him, then left. Emotionally, this felt like the beginning of the end for me—my self-confidence and hope began rapidly eroding.

Things went downhill very quickly at that point. One night, in the early morning hours, I woke up and realized that my bed was soaked. I had totally lost control—I was lying in a puddle of my own urine. When I tried to sit up, I could only get so far. Then something happened that made me feel like I was being crushed in a vise. I've since learned it's a condition called "MS banding" but at the time, I didn't know what the hell it was. I screamed out in pain.

Stephanie ran into the room, her eyes wide and scared. I looked at her at the foot of my bed and there were two of her. I just started crying. I thought, "She's not a twin. Which one of her is real?"

"Mommy?" she said, scared. "Mommy, what's wrong?"

Stephanie's school had just taught her how to call 911 and memorize an important number. I gasped out, "Sweetie, go call Papa. Call Papa."

My dad came over. "We've got to get you to a doctor," he said to me. "A new doctor. You need to see someone who can help figure out what's going on."

Off we went to see the second neurologist—me hopping on one leg and my dad dragging me along. The doctor worked at a leading medical institution in the San Francisco Bay Area. Once we got into the room, I explained some of the symptoms I'd been having. "I'm losing bladder control," I said. "I can't take care of my kid—which is my number one focus, I can't take care of my daughter." My voice caught and my eyes teared up. I took a breath and continued, keeping my voice calm. "I'm exhausted. I see two of everything. I have blind spots. My foot doesn't work. My leg doesn't work. I can't walk. I've lost my job." I paused. "My friends have been reading up on some of these symptoms and one of them mentioned that it could be multiple sclerosis, which is why I'm here."

"Could it be MS?" my dad asked.

The doctor raised his eyebrows skeptically. "MS is an extremely rare disease. Only 400,000 people in the entire country have MS." He paused, as if to let the impressiveness of this remark sink in. "I'm certain you do not have MS."

"Then, what is wrong with me?" I asked. "Why is my twenty-nine-year-old body failing me? I was fine a couple of months ago."

The doctor did a routine exam: He tested my reflexes. He looked into my ears. He checked my temperature. He listened to my lungs with a stethoscope. Then, he left the room.

Finally, he poked his head back into the room. "Why don't you join me in my office," he said to my dad and me. This was easier said than done. I couldn't do more than hobble, so my dad largely carried me back into the doctor's office.

We sat down. The doctor did not look at me. He did not address me. He never called me by my name. That was the first time in my entire life that I was *persona non grata*. Even when he glanced my way, he looked through me—like I was a ghost.

He spoke to my dad. "I don't think there is anything physically wrong with your daughter," he said decisively. "However, I do think she's very ill." As if to prove the point to my dad, he turned toward me and asked a series of bizarre questions: "Let me ask you some questions. Do you own a firearm?"

"No," I said, confused.

"Would you hurt yourself or your daughter?"

Both my dad and I were taken aback. The question seemed so bizarrely random. "No," I said, confused.

"What are you saying?" my dad asked.

He spoke again to my dad. "Do you think she would ever hurt herself or her daughter?"

I spoke louder. "NO!"

He continued speaking to my dad, ignoring me. "For example, would she jump off the Golden Gate Bridge?"

"NO!" I cried.

The doctor sighed. "Mr. Snow, I don't think there is anything physically wrong with your daughter. I think this is a severe form of mental illness. Her symptoms are manifestations of her mental illness." My dad and I stared at him in disbelief, both stunned. The doctor continued. "Since she's over the age of eighteen, I would encourage you to get her to sign this paperwork, so she can voluntarily go to a locked mental health facility for a seventy-two-hour evaluation."

I was reeling. I said, "I'm not crazy! I can't be in an institution! Who is going to raise my daughter?" He shrugged, which almost felt like a veiled threat—as if to say, "If you don't have anyone to mind your daughter, she can go to social services." I tried to shove down the rage and panic that was boiling up. My voice shook, but I tried to control it. I said, "I believe you're wrong."

"Well, I disagree with you," he said, his voice clipped. I felt like he had kicked me in the gut. I was so afraid, so scared—my fight or flight mode just exploded. That's when I sealed my fate with this guy, because I started screaming at him. Like "the crazy person" he accused me of being.

"Well, you know what?! FUCK YOU! I'm not crazy!" I yelled. "You're an asshole and I think you're the worst doctor I've ever seen!!" I pretty much screamed every obscenity combination I could think of.

My dad stood up and said, "Let's go." He helped support me to the car. I fell into the passenger seat, bawling my eyes out, my heart shattered.

Driving away, I would be lying if I didn't admit—for a moment—I wondered, "*Am* I crazy?" I had been taught to have faith in healthcare professionals and the institutions they work at. So far, the asshole and all my visits had only done one thing: let me down.

Now that I've spent over thirty years as a patient, navigating the healthcare world both for myself and countless others, I've realized my early experiences are not the norm. This book is not intended to be a bashing of the medical field in general. Thankfully, the majority of doctors are responsible and do not accuse patients of insanity as a first course of action. But in my case—he did. And the smug, white-coated authority of that doctor caused me to question everything. I *knew* these symptoms were real—but there was so much doubt put in me. Any self-esteem I'd had—any confidence or self-assuredness about my skills—was decimated. In an instant, it was like everything I had believed about myself simply vanished.

I *knew* these symptoms were real—but there was so much doubt put in me. In an instant, it was like everything I had believed about myself simply vanished.

I didn't know it at the time, but I was in the hellish throes of the first stage of the Patient's Journey: the fear, denial, pain, and desperate information seeking of the Pre-Diagnosis stage.

CONFUSION, DENIAL, AND DREAD

In the Pre-Diagnosis stage, you're dealing with a mixture of denial and fear. Weird things are happening to your body. You're getting tests done and it's scary waiting for the results to come in—the biopsy results, the breast exam, the blood test. There's a lot of fear. You might even have idiot doctors try to convince you that you're crazy.

People often use denial as a way to cope—both patients and their care partners: "There's nothing to worry about. It's probably nothing." You do a lot of self-talk in this stage. Sometimes, people do so much self-talk to push their fear down that they put off addressing the issue altogether. They prolong this stage by ignoring the symptoms as long as possible because they don't want to deal with the scary reality of what it might mean.

But that's the *worst* way to engage the Pre-Diagnosis stage. You need to work through that fear right out of the gate, because you've got to consider the end game: You want to live a life of meaning and impact. You want to have hope, and you don't want to limit your choices. The best thing you can possibly do for your future prospects is to get yourself checked out as soon as possible and try to figure out what's going on. If it walks like a duck, sounds like a duck, and smells like a duck—it's probably a duck. If you've got a pretty good idea that something's going wrong, denial will not be your friend. It will only make your Patient's Journey ten times harder.

In the Pre-Diagnosis stage, if you've got a pretty good idea that something's going wrong, denial will not be your friend. The best thing you can possibly do for your future prospects is to get yourself checked out as soon as possible and try to figure out what's going on.

The Ostrich Approach Is a Bad One

Many people in the Pre-Diagnosis stage instinctively know that there's something wrong—perhaps even dreadfully wrong—but they don't want to address it. They don't want to entertain the idea that the lump in their breast is potentially cancerous, so they wave it off as a random cyst that will probably go away. Or they ignore the mole on their skin that looks different. They make up an excuse for why they can't feel their left foot or hold a cup of water. Up to a certain point, many, many symptoms can be excused away. They can be excused away for a long time—right up to the point when all the wheels fall off the cart.

But taking the ostrich approach is a bad one, and here's why. There's *valuable time lost* when you're ignoring your body's warning signs. Every chronic illness and potentially terminal condition have something in common: the *earlier* you get diagnosed, the *better* your outcome. Period. End of discussion. This is a universal fact. That's why you want to get diagnosed as early as you can.

There's *valuable time lost* when you're ignoring your body's warning signs. The *earlier* you get diagnosed, the *better* your outcome. Get diagnosed as early as you can.

I know some people will read this and blow it off, because you're positive it's not going to happen to you. That's why I'm going to scare you a little with a cautionary tale. I want your story to take a different direction.

Recently, I was talking to a patient who'd had an abnormal pap smear. She went on the internet, looking for information that would make her feel better, and found articles about false positives. She concluded, "It's not a big deal. It's just a misreading." She didn't go to the follow-up appointment. She pushed the scary thoughts away, telling herself, "Abnormal pap smears happen to every woman. I'm probably completely fine."

Over a year later, she started having stomach pains and cramping up her back. Finally, she went back to the doctor. They asked her why she never came back for her follow up appointment. "This would have been good to catch much earlier. Things have progressed to a critical point."

A year and a few months after that abnormal pap smear, she now had stage four cervical cancer. It had metastasized to her liver, and her diagnosis was now poor.

These are the examples and the statistics you desperately want to avoid.

If you *have* ignored symptoms for all the understandable reasons you would want to, don't waste time beating yourself up about it. Simply focus on doing the best thing for yourself right now: pick up the phone and make a doctor's appointment. Best case scenario: it's a minor thing, and now you've gained peace of mind. If it's a worst case scenario and you *do* have a serious condition, there are even more reasons to make that appointment. The sooner you can get yourself answers, the sooner you can begin your healing journey.

If you have ignored symptoms for all the understandable reasons you would want to, don't waste time beating yourself up about it. Simply focus on doing the best thing for yourself right now: pick up the phone and make a doctor's appointment.

But it's not just your own denial that needs to be overcome—it's also the denial your closest people may be inclined to engage in. Listen: *no one* wants to believe you're very sick. Everyone would prefer to think your strange symptoms are a fluke or a trick of the mind: "You seemed to have a good day yesterday. How come you can't rise to the occasion today?" That inclination may come from a place of love, but it can put added pressure on you to advocate for the reality of your experience, even as you're struggling to keep it together while feeling so ill.

Some people may be even less charitable. If you don't have a black-and-white, cut and dry diagnosis confirming that you have a nameable disease, many people around you might be dismissive. Your absences at work might be chalked up to laziness, rather than legitimate health needs. If—God forbid—you urinate in the changing room, people assume you *elected* to do that and call you out in disgust. These experiences can shake your self-confidence and cause you to question your own gut instincts about what might be happening in your body. All of these factors can add additional hurdles in seeking out a diagnosis.

There's a lot of confusion in the Pre-Diagnosis stage. In many ways, it feels easier to stay in denial because no one wants an earth shattering moment confirming you have a life-altering disease. But at the same time, you're not going to be able to have a successful outcome *until* you can move forward with a diagnosis.

My hypothesis is that I've been able to live as full a life as I've lived because I got diagnosed with MS quickly. I was lucky enough to start taking the first FDA-approved drug for relapsing MS within a year and took a multidisciplinary approach, implementing critical modalities that helped strengthen and heal me. Granted, it took me about four months from the onset of my symptoms to get a diagnosis, but that was warp speed in 1993. When I was dealing with my first symptoms, it was not uncommon for MS patients to have to wait years before getting a name for what was happening to their bodies. Looking back, my quick diagnosis made an incalculable difference to my well-being.

I strongly encourage you to fight the temptation of denial. Face reality so that you can get your healing journey started as soon as possible.

Self-Diagnosis Is Dicey, Too

On the opposite end of the spectrum from denial, you've got frenzied, anxious attempts to self-diagnose. You're punching symptoms into your phone, waiting for AI to tell you what you have—even if the internet's conclusions are completely off base. I see this tendency occurring especially in the younger patient population. We're so used to living in a sphere of instant information, looking to influencers or bots who seem to have all the answers; we feel confident that the internet will know best.

Now, on the one hand, researching your symptoms is a better approach than denial. More information is better than less information, and ideally, your internet searches will give you more pointed topics to discuss with your doctor. (Spoiler alert: my own diagnosis came after friends helped me research my symptoms and we realized it might be MS. However, the official diagnosis only came after numerous tests by medical professionals. *That's* when my Patient's Journey moved forward.)

If you don't take your findings to your doctor, the self-diagnosis approach becomes dangerous. Most conditions—especially rare or complex ones—have overlapping symptoms. Your "bot" might give you one diagnosis when you actually have something else. And then what? You might have a serious illness, but you go about your life with a sense of false security, assuming that you have a more minor condition. Alternately, I know a person who began canceling all her social plans because she had convinced herself that she had a rare disease—even though no doctor had ever confirmed it. Her self-diagnosis led her to cut herself off from aspects of life that contributed to her well-being before ever seeking out proper medical testing or consulting a healthcare professional.

The subsequent actions you might take with a self-diagnosis pile on the problems. You may attempt to self-medicate in ways that could actually harm you. You may stop your pursuit of an official medical diagnosis if you feel content that you've already found the answer, meaning you don't set up the medical help you need. There's also a "Boy who cried 'wolf'" danger here, because people will be even less inclined to take your description of symptoms seriously if they know you diagnosed yourself.

Self-diagnosing can be especially problematic if you're struggling with your mental health. In the post-pandemic world, mental health struggles are widely prevalent. However, this is a particular area where outside objectivity is necessary for you to get the help you need. Mental illness is a real thing when it's a real thing. It's not okay to minimize it or to suggest that there is no such thing as psychosomatic symptoms or mental illness. Professional counselors, doctors, and therapists can help identify real occasions of mental illness and work with you to get on the right medication, if needed.

The outcome of both the denial approach and the self-diagnosis approach, ironically, is the same: You stall out. You can't move forward in your Patient's Journey. You can't get the services you need. You don't get help.

The outcome of both the denial approach and the self-diagnosis approach, ironically, is the same: you stall out on your Patient's Journey.

While there are many conditions that don't have medications or cures, there are many that *do*. Seeking out a correct diagnosis can ensure you get the proper care for your condition. If you self-diagnose in this stage because you don't want to go get a legitimate diagnosis for whatever reason, you will keep yourself in limbo, turning on a never-ending hamster wheel.

Push past your denial. Push past your fear. In the Pre-Diagnosis stage, the best thing you can do for yourself is to seek out the proper care you need.

HUNTING DOWN THE CORRECT DIAGNOSIS

Unfortunately, that's easier said than done.

You're sick. You're tired. Your self-esteem is shot. People don't believe you. Even when you muster up the courage to call doctors, you may find yourself on the shitty carousel I was on, going around in circles from doctor to doctor, getting a series of different diagnoses—none of which may actually be correct. You may be tempted to give up and never get to a place where you get a real answer. You're simply too sick and tired to keep trying.

So, how do you keep pushing for the diagnosis you need?

Here's my advice: you need to channel any intrinsic motivation you've got left to get a good answer. The hard fact of the matter is that, without a diagnosis for what's happening to you, you have almost no ability to pursue healing or craft a worthwhile life on the other side of illness. Your body will continue to suffer, your world will continue to contract, and your relationships will continue to experience tension.

So, do everything you can to muster up your intrinsic motivation to hunt that diagnosis. You might find new wells of motivation in yourself by considering your loved ones. We can often muster energy and bravery for others when we can't do it for ourselves—and that was certainly my story, as I'll share at the end of this chapter. Take a breather, regroup, and then *keep trying* until you get an answer that makes sense. Convince yourself that you need this more than anything else in your life right now—which is true. Lean on your friends, family, and partner if you need to. Get some trusted people to help you make those phone calls and drive you to appointments.

Embrace some bravado as you're hunting for your diagnosis. It takes chutzpah to demand better assessments than you may have initially gotten. You need gumption to say, "I deserve an answer." So, as much as you can, adopt that bravado! Push for the tests. Ask for a second opinion. You may have to go to twenty doctors before you get this figured out but *keep pushing* to figure out what's wrong. You matter.

Remember: my symptoms were first credited to sleep deprivation, a pinched nerve, postpartum issues, migraines, and psychosis before they were *finally* correctly diagnosed as MS. You also need that correct diagnosis. No forward movement can happen until you've got it. So, seek out a second or third or even fourth opinion if you need to. Pay attention to your body. And pay attention to your gut instinct. When you've heard three or four different opinions on what's happening to you, you'll know which one is right.

There will be many moments further into your Patient's Journey where you can be flexible, such as choosing a treatment or preferred therapeutic medication. But in the Pre-Diagnosis stage, you need to be inflexible about this. There is only one right way to move forward. You need the correct diagnosis.

There is only one right way to move forward in this stage:
you need the correct diagnosis.

MESSAGE TO CARE PARTNERS:
NAVIGATING PRE-DIAGNOSIS

If you are the partner of someone in the Pre-Diagnosis stage, the best thing you can do is validate what they're telling you about feeling ill. Don't give in to the temptation to indulge denial and tell them everything is sure to be okey-dokey. You can okey-dokey people to death. Instead, support your person by taking them seriously and showing that you care.

And keep in mind that "supporting" your person doesn't just mean patting them on the back and reassuring them that it's probably nothing. It's easy for partners to take the path of least resistance, but the best thing you can do for your sick someone is encourage them to seek out medical attention. Tell them, "Hey, stop scaring yourself on WebMD. You need to go see a doctor."

You might feel like you're being a hard-ass in those moments, especially if you get pushback from your person. You might feel like you're antagonizing them, rather than being their teammate. But if your sick person isn't showing a willingness, inclination, or the energy to be Team Captain—*you* need to help serve that role.

Gently, lovingly, help them get the diagnosis they need to move their journey forward. You can do that in a way that isn't antagonistic. Try saying, "I know you've been stressed and not feeling well. Why don't you let me make that appointment for you?" That's very different from saying, "You're not doing a damn thing for yourself, so I'm taking this into my own hands!" Same outcome, but two totally different approaches. Choose the one that helps you maintain the health of your relationship. The last thing you want to do is alienate your sick loved one, because you're going to need each other on this Patient's Journey.

ADVICE ON YOUR RESEARCH

In the quest for a correct diagnosis, you're going to be asking a lot of questions, consulting medical professionals, and doing your own digging. Here's a tip in that process: avoid what's not productive and ruthlessly pursue what *is* productive.

Here's what's *not* productive: going down internet rabbit holes that detail all the ways your symptoms equate certain death. Physicians who blow off your concerns or want to suggest a superficial solution. Your own head in the sand.

Here's what *is* productive: gleaning key points from research that you can discuss with your doctor. Asking for tests. Working with medical professionals who take you seriously, order the *right* tests, and demonstrate a genuine desire to help you get to the bottom of what's going on.

In the Pre-Diagnosis stage, you could easily invite a massive deluge of information: facts about various diseases related to your symptoms, research articles, new Google searches, terrifying anecdotal stories from friends, and so on. All of that can be overwhelming and stir up huge fear. It can also, disastrously, cause you to become so discouraged that you stop seeking a diagnosis.

So, in this early stage of your illness, I recommend you *only take in as much as you are emotionally and mentally able to handle.* Three decades ago, when I was starting my own Patient's

Journey, there was no search engine called Google, but my friends and family were doing research for me about MS. They would drop off books from the public library for me to read, and I'd be staring at chapter titles like, "Multiple Sclerosis: The Crippler of Young Adults." I'd see statistics that practically guaranteed I'd be living in a wheelchair for the rest of my life. And that was way too intense for me, initially. It was beyond depressing, totally overwhelming, and too much for me to handle at that time.

A lack of information is certainly a bigger problem than too much information. But you may have to find ways to skim through it, so you get everything that's relevant for your decision-making, while still protecting yourself from information that's upsetting, counterproductive, unhelpful, or distracting.

If there's one area to prioritize in this initial research, it's gathering information about *who* is going to treat you and *how* you're going to be treated. You need to find the right doctor who will take you seriously, validate your concerns, and ideally, determine correctly what's going on with your body. The right physician will also help determine your treatment protocols, required tests, and so on.

The most important area to research is gathering information about *who* is going to treat you and *how* you're going to be treated. You need to find the right doctor who will take you seriously, validate your concerns, and ideally, determine correctly what's going on with your body.

Until that piece is in place, everything else needs to be on hold. You need to get the right medical care established if you hope to move forward on this Journey into greater health. Maintain the tenacity to keep pushing for a correct diagnosis. Keep seeking the answers you need. Fight to get a name for what's happening to you. And if you can't do it for yourself—do it for the people you love.

CARE PARTNER PERSPECTIVE: MARA L.

"Are you home yet? Call me when you get there." My dad's words cut through the chilly New York City fall air and I knew in my gut that something was not right. It was Halloween night. I was twenty-three, fresh out of school and embarking on my new adult life in the city.

When I got home to my tiny studio apartment, I called my dad back and heard the words: "I have cancer." *I. Have. Cancer.* My world stopped and my head spun. How could this have happened? How did we get here? Would he die? How would I survive without him? Through my tears I heard him tell me that he had been feeling sick with a virus he couldn't shake. At first, he'd brushed it off—he was a locally renowned pediatrician, so he was surrounded by germs all the time. He had finally gone to his PCP who suspected there was something more going on, leading to a diagnosis of angioimmunoblastic T-cell lymphoma. The prognosis was shockingly grim.

The next weeks were blurry with tears, plane flights and life-changing decisions. I found myself resigning my brand-new teaching position and moving back home, jobless, not knowing what was ahead for my family. However, though I knew that we were about to be forever changed, I didn't know that my life's brightest moments would come from that point of darkness. All the best parts of my life were born from the night I learned of his diagnosis. I know that is the legacy he left for me.

"STAY POSITIVE. STAY POSITIVE."

After the Asshole Physician told my dad and me that I should be committed to a mental institution, I was not doing well. I collapsed into the passenger seat of my dad's car, sobbing.

My dad was gripping the steering wheel, staring out the windshield as he accelerated down the onramp. "You've just gotta stay positive, Bren," he said. "Stay positive. Stay positive. It will get better."

Stay positive. That's the closest thing to a Snow Family Credo we've got. I'd heard that phrase my entire life, and for most of my life, I believed it. But at that time, it was the last fucking thing I wanted to hear. If my left arm had been working, I would have given dear old dad a good smack.

I didn't feel positive. I didn't see how anything could or would get better. I stayed silent while my dad repeated those words. And as soon as I got home, I gave up.

My dad left to go pick up Stephanie from school, leaving me alone. I lay there in bed, thinking, *Well, this is it. This is my future. I'm going to be a disabled person. I probably won't be able to do anything for myself. I won't be able to take care of Stephanie.*

My thoughts kept spiraling down, and down, and down. I concluded that life was cruel. Other than my daughter, I had nothing to live for. I thought bleakly, *I'll just try to put on a stupid, brave face for her.* But even as I tried to muster up the will to make that decision, I gave up hope in having a happy life. I had no hope in anything. I was gutted to my soul.

And I was still scared—I still didn't even know what I had. Was it *cancer*? I didn't know.

Finally, I put myself out of my misery by letting the crippling fatigue of MS put me to sleep.

Normally, when Stephanie got home, I'd be there to greet her. I couldn't that day; I was too sick to do anything but lie in bed. She came and found me and asked, "Mommy?" I opened my eyes and looked at her bleakly. I couldn't do anything. I didn't *want* to do anything, either. I lay there, lifeless. Her big blue eyes got wide and scared. Tears started coming down her little face. She said, "Mommy, are you going to die?" She sounded so afraid.

I didn't know how to answer her question. *Was* I going to die? I didn't know. But as I looked at her, I thought, *I'm all she has.*

She had only just begun to think about those big questions about life and death. And now, it was *my* death that was looming as a possibility in her mind.

Some courageous part of me spoke up in my brain. *She's YOURS. And she needs you. And you will do anything—to your last breath—to be there for her. She fucking deserves better than what you're giving her right now. She deserves more.*

I closed my eyes, willing the brave part of me to get stronger. *I have to show strength. I cannot let her feel that she's going to be abandoned, or alone, or that she's not going to have a parent. I've got to do everything I can to keep fighting for her.*

Slowly, I pushed myself up to sit. I took a deep breath and looked at my daughter. "I'm not going to die," I said to her. "But I'm very sick. I don't know what's wrong with me." She climbed into the bed and curled into me.

Only an hour before, I had decided to give up on doctors and resign myself to this being my destiny. But as I looked at Stephanie, I thought, *This is not the example I want to set for her. I don't WANT to give up.*

Within the next twenty-four hours, I got a hold of my dad. "I need to go to one more doctor," I told him.

I had to keep trying. I needed a name for what was happening to me. I needed a diagnosis.

STAGE 1 OF THE PATIENT'S JOURNEY: PRE-DIAGNOSIS

- *Common emotions: fear, confusion, denial, anxious self-diagnosing.*
- *Common pitfalls: ignoring symptoms and hoping they'll go away, convincing yourself there's nothing wrong, diagnosing yourself incorrectly and failing to seek out medical attention, despair.*
- *Your best next step: Get checked out! Don't rest until you get an answer for what's happening to your body.*

CHAPTER 3

Diagnosis

LEVERAGE THE POWER OF CONNECTIVITY TO RIDE
OUT AN IDENTITY EARTHQUAKE

"You are not judged by the height you have risen, but from the depth you have climbed."

— Frederick Douglass

The journey to a diagnosis can be brutal and cause you to question your own sanity. If and when a diagnosis finally comes, there can be some relief—since, thank goodness, there's finally a *name* for what's happening to you—but there's also fear. You're confronted with questions you never wanted to consider: "What does this mean? What kind of future is in front of me now? How does this change things? How does this change *me?*"

Most challenging of all, getting diagnosed with a chronic or terminal illness can usher in an identity earthquake. Pivotal parts of your identity like your physical appearance, your career, your contribution to your family—basically, your ability to *do* things— are all called into question as you are given a new label: a sick person.

But by strengthening your connection to others and your self-connection, you can reclaim your identity in the midst of the Diagnosis stage. Although it will be challenging, it's crucial to trust your instincts and stand confidently on what you know to be true. This will only help you as the going gets rough, and it'll help pave the way for a profound transformation.

By strengthening your connection to others and your self-connection, you can reclaim your identity in the midst of the Diagnosis stage.

FINDING FIRMER GROUND: A DIAGNOSIS

In December 1993, I went and saw another neurologist—the first female doctor I'd seen since my symptoms began. She *listened* to me. And then she conducted a full neurological examination.

We started with an Ishihara vision test, which tested me for optic neuritis—a possible telltale symptom of MS. She showed me a book that had a circle made up of lots of little dots in different colors. She said, "What do you see there?"

I looked at her, confused. In my mind, I thought, *I don't see shit.* Out loud, I said, "I see dots."

"Do you see a number here?"

I stared at the circle. "No. Nothing." Was I *supposed* to be seeing colors and number patterns? I felt a slow buildup of alarm.

There were other neurological tests that examined my reflexes: my doctor asked me to close my eyes and touch my nose. I couldn't touch my nose. She asked me to wiggle my toes and move my ankle. Couldn't do that. She ran a pin up my foot and said, "Tell me when you feel something." I didn't feel anything but tried telling myself it might just be because she wasn't pressing hard enough. Then, she went to my other side and repeated the process. I thought, *Well, shit, I can feel something over there.*

With each test, I was intellectualizing the fact that things were not going well. On the one hand, I appreciated that this doctor wasn't just sending me away with a prescription for headache medicine. On the other hand, I quickly began to see that something was rotten in the state of Brenda.

At the end of the examination, my doctor put her hand on my shoulder and said, "Ms. Snow." Instantly, my eyes filled with tears. Her kindness, coupled with the fact that she was the first doctor to show me the respect of calling me by my name, was nearly overwhelming. I finally felt like I was being treated as a human being— not a hysterical person making things up in my head.

But I also wept because I knew she was about to tell me something awful. Deep down, what I had known to be true from day one was about to become reality.

She said, "I don't think you're crazy. But I do think that you are very sick. And I think you quite possibly have multiple sclerosis. What we need to do is send you to the hospital for a lumbar puncture and an MRI to confirm that suspicion."

There it was: a name. A diagnosis. And one I would have never, ever chosen. I knew that MS was a shit thing to get, and I had never wanted to hear the words "multiple sclerosis" applied to me, just like nobody ever wants to hear they have cancer. But at the same time, I felt a sense of relief and validation. Somewhere in the recesses of my mind, I thought, *Well, if it has a name, maybe I can get some damn help.*

Within a few hours, I was admitted to the hospital. I went down for an MRI the first day, and the next morning, I endured the lengthy and painful lumbar puncture. That evening, my doctor made her rounds and came into my room. I registered the fact that she did *not* come in and cheerfully announce, "Good news!"

Instead, she sat on the edge of my bed, looked at me kindly, and spoke with gentle firmness. "Ms. Snow, we have the results of your testing. We see some oligoclonal bands in your cerebral spinal fluid. We can also see a small lesion in your cerebellum. This is confirming, along with your clinical examination, the diagnosis of multiple sclerosis."

I had the strange sensation of trying to make up my mind about whether or not it was the worst day of my life or the best day of my life. On the one hand, this was the day I'd been told I had MS, an incurable, debilitating chronic illness. On the other hand, I had finally been validated by the healthcare community that this illness was real, which might mean I could finally start dealing with these symptoms.

In between bleak thoughts of a destroyed future, I thought, *Hell. If there's a name for it, I'm going to figure it out. Because I'm not going to stay like this. I'm going to find a way to get better.*

RELIEF AND FEAR

Most patients—me included—feel a mixture of relief and fear in the moment they get a diagnosis. On the one hand, it's validating. Some well-educated medical person confirms what you've suspected: "You have cancer. That's why you're experiencing so much pain." "You have multiple sclerosis. You're not crazy." Once there's a label, you can officially get help. Insurance coverage kicks in. You can get the right doctors a seat at the table. You can line up your specialists and all the therapeutics you might need to start a treatment and hopefully begin building toward a new normal. But it's also a very frightening moment. It confirms the fears you may have been pushing aside. I thought, *If it has a name, I can do something about it.* But at the same time, I was like, *What the fuck, are you joking? How is this my life?*

The Diagnosis stage brings both relief and depression. You look for someone to blame and feel overwhelmed by all the information you need to take in.

The Diagnosis stage can also cause you to feel seriously shaken in your identity. One day, you're a healthy person and the next day, you have a *label.* That's why one of the most important ways to care for yourself in this stage is to hold on to the precious, truest parts of who you are through one of the most earth-shattering experiences of your life: getting diagnosed with a terrible disease.

IDENTITY EARTHQUAKE
I'm originally from California, and I have experienced powerful earthquakes when the ground beneath you starts shaking and cracking. *That's* the sensation of suddenly realizing you're a person with a disease. The diagnosis feels like an earthquake. The foundation feels broken. There are cracks in the walls. You feel like all the skills that you've developed and honed from your infancy are suddenly irrelevant. Your sense of confidence and identity is massively altered because it's like, "Wait a second—I'm a *sick person.*"

What does that mean? What happens to your identity or self-worth when you're a sick person? It can easily feel like you've suddenly transformed into this *thing* that needs to do these other *things* if you want to get well or save your life. You feel subhuman, somehow. The impact on your identity is mind blowing. I asked myself, "Does this mean I'm still Brenda? How can I be Brenda if I can't do the things that Brenda does?"

A diagnosis can feel like an earthquake.

It's not hard to understand why the next stage in the Patient's Journey is Grief. Very quickly, a deep sadness sweeps in from the perceived loss of your sense of self, your confidence, what you're able to accomplish, and even your personality. If you don't feel well or you have to sleep all the time or take mood-altering medications—those things all affect your sense of self.

And the identity earthquake, unfortunately, can be reinforced by other people—even well-meaning people. They say things like, "Oh, you don't seem so good." "Gosh, sorry—you look terrible." "Are you sure you're okay?" They're trying to validate you, but their comments can make your efforts to get back to center feel like running on a hamster wheel. The message that gets reinforced is, "Now, you're a *patient.*"

Yes, you're a patient.

You're also *still you*.

In this chapter, I want to help you stay tightly connected to *you* during the Diagnosis phase. Stay grounded, first of all, in the fact that the identity earthquake is normal.

You don't feel normal. Your whole world has just been jolted with a magnitude 9.0 earthquake. But what you're experiencing *is normal* for every patient. This is part of it.

Now, what can you do to successfully ride out the identity earthquake? Lean into the power of connectivity: build up your connection to others, and build up—especially—your self-connection.

The Power of Connectivity

Two or three months into my diagnosis, I found myself trying to survive by leaning into connectivity. I was innately strengthening my connection to my own personality and what I wanted from my life, and I was also leaning into connections with my friends and family. I wasn't naming that connectivity as a tool or even thinking about the fact that I was doubling down on strengthening those ties. It just felt like a necessary means of survival.

The irony was while, as a person and a social being, I identified connectivity as a powerful way to keep my shit together, the exact opposite of that was going on inside my body. MS is a demyelinating disease; it degrades the neural connection between brain and body. The myelin sheath protects nerves as they run from the brain and spinal cord to the rest of the body; basically, it facilitates the brain's messages to the rest of your body to keep it working properly. If you think of your nerves as wires, the myelin sheath can be imagined like the insulation around those wires. Multiple sclerosis creates lesions on the myelin sheath. And wherever a lesion forms, there's a corresponding breakdown of communication between that exposed nerve and whatever other body part it's supposed to be sending messages to. That's why my left leg had stopped working.

And why my eyes sometimes saw double. That's why I was having trouble controlling my bladder: demyelination. The connections were breaking down.

But in some strange way, my body's demyelination became a driver for me. I had a disease that was causing the connections within my own body to unravel: I looked different, couldn't walk, and couldn't do things I used to do. As a result, I resolved that I had to remember who I really was and what I was all about. I had to double down on my "self-connection": my personal headline, my core values, and my gut feelings. I had to strengthen connections to my main people and build new connections with members of my health team. I had a demyelinating disease, but I was strengthening the connections in every other part of my life. I wasn't about to let *everything* unravel.

In the Diagnosis stage, strengthen your connection to others and your connection to self.

And this was a game changer for me. By strengthening my connections to others and myself, I navigated the scary part of my diagnosis with a strong grip on my identity and the people I loved. I've watched many other patients successfully ride out the identity earthquake by similarly leaning into their community and keeping their grip on deeper aspects of their identity—ones that can't easily be shaken, even by disease.

Some people reading this book will be coming to the table with a strong, tightly knit community already. Some people will already have a strong sense of self, starting their Patient's Journey with a lot of confidence and stability.

Other patients navigating this journey are more fragile. They don't have as strong a sense of self, confidence, or self-esteem. They might have a background of trauma, prolonged stress, or adverse childhood experiences. Getting a chronic or serious diagnosis can trigger a huge added weight. It's incredibly easy to go straight to, "Why me? Why me when I've already suffered so much?" When you put a grave illness on top of someone coming in with past injuries, it can feel like the straw that breaks the camel's back. For all those reasons, the strategies I'm going to recommend may feel more challenging for people who fall in this category—*but they're also that much more important.*

You can think of your ability to connect to yourself and others in terms of structures in an earthquake. A structure that was built on a strong foundation with solid construction will get through an earthquake with a lot less damage than a house built with shaky walls on uneven ground.

So—what do we do with those more fragile structures? We build them up. They need extra support. They need attention and maintenance.

What are specific steps you can take to embrace this power of connectivity during the Diagnosis stage? I'll talk first about connecting to others and then outline ways you can shore up your even more essential connection to self.

CONNECTING TO OTHERS

Whether or not you're starting out with a strong community, it's incredibly important for you to *get connected* to others, even when it's the last thing you feel like doing. Let's talk about two key ways to do that.

Shore Up Community

In a perfect world, you're entering this Diagnosis phase with a circle of supportive family and friends. If that's not your situation, then start finding your people by asking your healthcare team for leads. There are many types of support groups and ways to get connected—lbut you'll need to make an effort to search them out. Your healthcare providers might also be able to point you toward local support groups or even national advocacy organizations that do virtual meetings, round tables, and discussions. Finding a group of other people you can connect with is a far better use of your time online than reading a bad blog. Local groups are even better. You might be able to find one that's disease specific.

Also, don't be afraid to reach out for services. There are many services—locally, statewide, and federally—that can help provide basic necessities, resources, and companionship. Additionally, one place I see many patients finding support is through faith-based organizations. Whether you are a spiritual person or not, a faith-based community may be helpful in surrounding you with love and support. They are there in service and—more often than not—these communities are where you may meet supportive people. The same principles apply to community and civic organizations. At the end of the day, people really do want to help. You just have to take the first step—even if you can't walk.

Now, I will say this: when you feel like garbage, it's hard to have the energy to seek these communities out, let alone engage with them. But a little effort will go a long way. Think through the people in your orbit. There is probably *somebody* in your life—whether it's your friend, a doctor, a nurse, a work colleague, or whomever—who would eagerly help get you plugged in. You have to be a hand raiser. And if you can't do it, you must ask somebody else to help you get connected.

Be a hand raiser. Or, if you don't have the energy to do it yourself, ask somebody else to help you get connected.

Trusted Confidant

Among your community of people, you'll fare especially well if you have *your* person: a trusted confidant—someone who can handle your TMI, laugh at your crabbiness, and help you remember who you really are. This might be your care partner, but ideally, you'll have more than one confidant. Your care partner will often need time for themselves to process and sort through the huge changes this diagnosis is bringing to *their* life, as well. Both of you will benefit from the support of a trusted friend who won't be scared off by oxygen tubes, walking sticks, cancer wigs, or ugly crying.

My Aunt Melinda was this person for me. I verbalized to her early in the days after I got my diagnosis, "I need you to tell me that I haven't changed. At least not in the ways that count. Tell me my sense of humor is still intact. Tell me I'm still *me*."

Later in the hospital, I was put on a very high dose of IV steroids. That meant I would get unbelievable cravings and had an enormous appetite. Basically, I could eat for twelve. I once told Melinda, "I need a taco." She went to Taco Bell and brought us back a twelve-pack of tacos. She thought we were going to share the twelve tacos as she climbed into the hospital bed with me, but I think I ate them all! We both started laughing. She said to me at that moment, "See?! You're your same self. You still love tacos! You haven't changed."

When I told Melinda how I had yelled at the jerk doctor, she laughed again. "Ha! You don't have to worry about losing yourself. You're still a ballbuster!" She was my bestie, and I'm so glad that I asked her to please remind me along the way about *me*, because she was able to do that.

Enormous power can come from identifying a safe, trusted, nonjudgmental confidant who can stand there and say, "You've got this." This person can serve as a touchstone to remind you—even if you feel like you've changed—they can still see the glimmers of who you are.

MESSAGE TO CARE PARTNERS: DEALING WITH PERSONALITY CHANGES

It's not uncommon for patients to have a temporary change in personality, either because of their symptoms or their medications. "Chemo brain" is a real thing, for instance, which may cause some cancer patients to have mental fog or not feel like themselves. In my case, the intense steroids I was put on to deal with my inflammation caused an increase in anger and irritability. Usually, these personality changes will only last as long as the treatment, but there are also other changes to expect due to the disease's symptoms. For example, fatigue, sadness, irritability—those all may be par for the course in patients as they grapple with painful physical changes.

You have two objectives in the midst of all this: 1) help remind your loved one who they truly are, and 2) care for yourself.

Many of the strategies I'll go on to discuss in this chapter are ones you can help lead your loved one in; for instance, creating a memory book with pictures that help the patient remember who they are at their core, or helping them identify their personal headline. Also, it's important for you to remember to be empathetic with your loved one's limitations. Pushing them to do deep identity work may be too big of an ask on any given day. Sometimes your loved one will simply need your comfort and love, without being pushed to do anything else. Other times, they may be in a headspace to do some of the important identity work we talk about in this chapter, and that's when you can help bring them along to shore up their connection to self.

Also, care for yourself. This is especially important in cases where a patient's diagnosis causes a *permanent* change in personality, as in the case of a cognitive disorder like Alzheimer's or a traumatic brain injury. In those cases, take full advantage of respite care to help you persevere. Give yourself breaks. It can be helpful for both care partners and patients to lean on other people. This helps "change the scenery" and introduces other empowering voices into your world, which can be a significant morale boost to you both.

Finally, lean on other friends, family, and community members to help remind *you* of who you really are. Their support is crucial for your own resilience and well-being. This experience is likely to be incredibly hard, but it will also allow you to grow in important, profound ways.

CONNECTING TO SELF

But what about your own self talk? What does it actually look like to experience this identity earthquake during the Diagnosis stage of the Patient's Journey?

It might mean huge insecurity—and again, that's normal. It's normal to totally lose your confidence and feel sad over the person you were. I remember looking in the mirror and not even recognizing myself. The intravenous steroids I was put on led to a weight gain of fifty pounds in a short timeframe. Sometimes, the changes from your illness can mean you literally don't recognize the person staring back at you in the mirror. There are weird, painful physical symptoms caused by your illness, which make you feel lost in your own body.

And the changes that occur inwardly are sometimes even more shocking. It's not uncommon to experience mood alterations, either from the pain of your symptoms or the medications you have to take. Cognitive changes are frequent: your thinking and memory may get foggy. It's also not uncommon to feel plagued by guilt. In my years of experience talking to thousands of patients, they often start with the questions, "Why did this happen to me? What did I do to deserve this? Is this a result of my choices or behaviors, somehow?" Almost everyone starts a self-punishing narrative. But while that might be normal, it's simply not reality: Nobody does anything to deserve a chronic condition. And damaging self-talk only adds pain to an already painful, confusing time.

That's why—as important as it is for you to connect with others—it's even more important for you to strengthen your connection with yourself. This disease will shake you to the core, but there are elements of your core that are unshakeable. When you identify what those are, you have something strong and solid to cling to. These strategies will help you find bedrock.

This disease will shake you to the core, but there are elements of your core that are unshakeable. When you identify what those are, you have something strong and solid to cling to.

Memory Book

Your first strategy for strengthening your self-connection is an easier one because—obviously—you're not feeling very well. This is a gentle place to start. We'll ramp up to the deep soul searching in a moment.

Keeping a journal is simple and easy to do, and it can be profoundly grounding. I don't say this flippantly, although the encouragement to journal is often thrown around in a flippant way. Keeping a journal can be incredibly beneficial down the road. I had no idea how beneficial it would be for me.

In the early days of my illness, I thought of my own journal as a "memory book." I had some cognitive impairment and memory loss early on, and my memory book was literally a strategy to help me remember important things. If I had the strength to write a sentence or a paragraph, I would do it. If I didn't, I'd ask someone to help me.

I did not do this eloquently. I did not use any particular prompts. It was mostly a stream of consciousness—something that would capture my pulse on any given day. I wrote down, "I'm worried about [this]. I'm stressed about [that]." It was not poetry. It was verbal vomit. And it felt better to get it out!

I also used my memory book as a way to help me heal. I had a cassette tape—that's how long ago it was—with guided visual imagery. The voice prompted me to "visualize my cells healing." In my mind, I imagined all my "bad disease cells" washing away. And then I imagined my stress and my fears washing away, and my insecurities washing away. It brought me back to who I was *going* to be, who I *wanted* to be. I did those guided imagery sessions every night before bed, and then I wrote down some of the helpful thoughts that came out of it in the memory book.

I wrote down my hopes and dreams. I got out my fears. I remembered who I was.

I probably wrote a lot of swear words down, too! (You are getting to know me.)

When I looked at the book again, I could see the disease was real. It was really happening to me—it wasn't just a bad dream. My own recorded data forced me to acknowledge it. And then, importantly, the entries in the book confirmed that I was *doing something about it*. I was taking action in necessary, important ways.

The book also helped banish some of the self-doubt that had been stirred up before I was diagnosed. It was evidence that I was *not* crazy. The self-doubt was very real and very big. But by tracking my disease's progress in the journal, I was deliberately processing to move myself forward. It was an act that helped me claim hope that I would be okay again one day.

I encourage you to do the same. By regularly capturing the state of your mind, body, and soul, you ensure that you're charting your sense of self, your hopes and dreams, and your fears. The result is an anchor to ground you and remind you of what's true.

Focus on the Wins

Another easy strategy: be deliberate about taking stock of the small bits of progress you're making. It might seem like you are making none at first—literally none—for the first several months you're living with your condition. But that's often because you're using a pre-diagnosis yardstick.

Here's what I mean by that. You can't say, "I used to be able to cook the meal at Christmas and I stayed up late and wrapped all the gifts. This Christmas, I was only able to stay awake for an hour. I'm such a loser." Stop that! You need to switch that thinking. Look at your *progress*. "Well, two weeks ago, I didn't even get out of bed. So, compared to that, being awake for an hour and seeing the kids open their gifts is … a win."

BAM. A *big* win. You've got to celebrate that! *That* is a powerful moment of connection to self.

I'm not trying to be the positivity poster girl here, but you have to reframe what good looks like. You have to reframe what *confidence* looks like. You need to use a new yardstick to measure the wins properly. If you're a patient undergoing chemo and radiation and you managed to sit through dinner with your family? That's a win. Did you brush your own teeth? WIN. Did you get to the bathroom and pee by yourself? *WINNING*. These are big, giant milestones, and claiming them as such can do wonders for your self-esteem.

Focus on those steps of progress and remember: You are still achieving things. You are still growing. *You are still awesome.*

Use a new yardstick to measure the wins properly.
Celebrate your progress!

Know Your Personal Headline

As you're staying connected to yourself, rediscovering what it means to live in your skin, and assimilating the grief, trauma, and fear of your diagnosis on the way to acceptance, it's worth facing some big questions, such as:

- How's my life going to look?
- What's my purpose that will guide my time, however long it lasts? This may crystallize for you at different junctures on your Patient's Journey. Early in my journey, my purpose was focused on getting better for Stephanie.
- What's the personal headline that can keep me grounded? Think of your personal headline as a brief short-term goal for yourself, or a confirmation of the identity *you* choose; for instance, "I am not defined by my disease."
- How can I let my personal headline *evolve* throughout these Patient Journey stages?

For me, early on, my personal headline was simply: "I won't feel like this forever. And one day, I'm going to walk again." I had three doctors say I wouldn't walk again, but I hung on to this personal mission. It was aspirational—but I knew that if I wanted to achieve anything, I needed to first acknowledge what that thing was, state it out loud, keep it top of mind, and not deviate from it, even with the infiltration of my disease.

Two years later, I had a very different personal headline, because I'd made it to a very different place. I *was* walking again, and I had made a lot of progress. So then, it was, "I'm going to do something to change patients' lives with my story."

My personal headline was a way to architect my journey. It was me "manifesting" before anyone called it that. The headline provided me with a roadmap of where I was going to direct my energy and effort.

Your personal headline is like your own mission statement. It's a way to architect your journey, providing you with a roadmap of where to direct your energy and effort.

Maybe you've put off this kind of reflection in the past, but there's nothing like a chronic or terminal illness to cause you to think about the purpose of your life. Lean into that. Identify the mission that will keep you moving forward, so you can choose decisions that reflect hope in your future.

Hang On to Your Core Values

Another strategy to help you strengthen your self-connection is to identify some of your core values. Once you enter the Diagnosis stage, there's a lot of incoming noise. So much information comes at you that you're lucky if you absorb 40 percent of it. Everybody's got an opinion. Everybody's trying to help. Noise, noise, noise.

In the midst of that, hold on to what you know to be true—or even what you *want* to be true. Your core values are the beliefs and choices that deeply connect to how you make all your decisions. They can help guide you as you navigate some of your hardest days.

In my family, staying positive was a value my parents held religiously. That was hard for me at first, because early on in my illness, I felt negative about 80 percent of the time. But during the 20 percent of the time I *didn't* feel like absolute hell, I would remember, "Dad promised me that good things happen when I stay positive. Everything looks better when I stay positive." And once I stopped hating all things that resembled a glass-half-full, I realized that I *had* to start using positivity to think differently about things.

Every obstacle—every hard, shitty thing I hated, I looked at and tried to reframe in a way where I could identify just a *little* bit of the upside. I hunted for just a *little* bit of positivity. I deliberately changed my self-talk: "I'm only thirty years old. I have a long life in front of me. MS isn't going to kill me—unless I keep this negative attitude, in which case, I'm going to waste my life feeling sorry for myself and I'm not going to make it past thirty-five." I'd been raised to value positivity. I was going to hang on to it to the bitter end.

Another core value that I held on to tightly was expertise. I had gotten quite a lot of poor counsel early on from healthcare providers who didn't look at my situation in its entirety. Even after my diagnosis, I was pitched "snake oil cures" and all kinds of bad science by people who claimed they wanted to help. I approached it all with skepticism. I didn't want a bogus diagnosis. I also didn't want false hope. I wanted information that was grounded in solid research and thoroughly peer reviewed. That value served me well and kept my head on straight.

And I held on to tenacity as a core value. I was determined to not give up, even on the days when I didn't feel well or was depleted of energy. It was challenging to keep fighting—exhausting, in fact. But I knew that when all was said and done, I was only going to get better through hard work and sticking with the therapies. I had to be tenacious in sorting through good and bad information. I had to be tenacious to keep working at getting better even when I wanted to give up. I had to be tenacious in choosing a positive mindset. That was the only way forward.

I've seen patients choose to claim the value that they're not alone—and I hope this book makes that value ring true. There are other people who have walked this road before you. There are people out there you don't even know yet who will come into your world and light it up with their inspirational words and actions. Knowing you're not alone—claiming that as a reality, and reaching out in kind—is incredibly powerful. Identify the values that pull your focus toward what is real and true and good. There's no shortage of noise and opinions and information coming your way right now. It can be easy to lose sight of your own self in the midst of all that. But by holding on to your core values, you keep yourself as the captain of the ship on your Patient's Journey.

Identify the values that pull your focus toward what is real and true and good. By holding on to your core values, you keep yourself as the captain of the ship on your Patient's Journey.

Trust Your Gut

Every one of us in life has an innate inner sense that guides our decision-making. Call it intuition or God's gift, call it the lessons we were taught—every one of us has that inner voice that pricks us when we make bad choices or pushes us to make good ones. It's your gut instinct—the voice inside you that points you toward truth. That inner truth can get diminished over time by our life choices, and it can also get diminished by disease.

I was so sick, my ability to listen to myself shriveled to the size of a little piece of corn. The asshole doctor told me I was crazy and suggested I might hurt my daughter, and I *almost* believed him. I would have—if I hadn't listened to my gut.

I *knew* I wasn't crazy. Even though that doctor decimated my confidence, I knew I would never, ever hurt my daughter. I knew I wouldn't harm myself. I didn't know much at that point, but I knew that.

You have to listen to your gut. Let that inner truth percolate up to the surface. It's easy to push it down and buy into the nonsense that since you didn't go to medical school, the jerk physician must know more than you. To hell with that. Seek out a second or third or even fourth opinion if you need to. Pay attention to your body. And pay attention to your gut instinct. In the Pre-Diagnosis stage, this was especially relevant: you had to be open to the idea that several doctors might have different opinions on what was happening to you, and decide which one you thought was right. It's relevant in the Diagnosis stage as well: as you hear different opinions on the best course of treatment, you may need to seek out a range of opinions on which next steps will work best for you.

Hone your ability to listen to yourself by doing the journaling, focusing on your wins, identifying your personal headline and your core values, and trusting your gut. All of those practices will help water that inner voice and allow it to flower. That strengthened connection to your inner voice will be one of the key things that propel you forward.

EARLY INFORMATION GATHERING

There's one last point I want to make about the Diagnosis stage of your Patient's Journey, and that's a heads up about the information gathering that will be required. Later in this book I've devoted an entire chapter to Optimizing Your Care, which will help guide you in actively seeking out information about the best therapeutics, providers, and so on. But there's an earlier phase of Information Gathering that happens now—and it's like drinking from a firehose. With your diagnosis comes *a lot of information.* And to some degree, you have to learn a new language to comprehend all the new terminology that's suddenly relevant to your survival. It can be overwhelming, so I want to give you some pointers to navigate the deluge:

- **You have all the right skills to learn what you need to learn.** Yes, it's confusing, but you will learn. You are smart. Just ask the questions you need answered. Don't worry about bothering the doctor—it's part of their job to answer your questions.
- **Lean into your friends and community for the help that you require.** If you can't handle all the information that's being shoved at you, farm it out. Ask for their help comprehending it all. Ask for their presence at doctor visits. Let them shoulder some of the load. Remember: connecting to others is now one of your survival skills.
- **Don't over-Google.** There's a healthy balance between "need to know" and over-information. There are also good sites with healthy information, and there are websites that are total garbage. *Monitor yourself* in the age where every bit of information is right at your fingertips. The right patient stories can be uplifting and inspirational, but there's also a lot of shit out there that will do the opposite. Be a wise information consumer.

- **Find a doctor who takes you seriously.** Sometimes, you start out with a "lemon doctor," who—like a lemon car—will clearly not take you very far. That happened to me, and I needed to find a new doctor. Especially if you have a chronic condition that you'll be dealing with for the rest of your life, you need to choose a doctor like you would choose a spouse. You don't want to be working with someone you can't stand or who won't give you the time of day. It behooves you to spend the time seeking out your best possible team. Find a doctor who is knowledgeable, skillful, takes good care of you, and makes you feel comfortable asking questions. If there's any part of you that thinks, "I don't want to bother the doctor"—that's a sign you need a new team. Otherwise, it's going to be a bumpy ride and lead you to questionable outcomes. Your doctor *should* give you access, they *should* explain things well, and they *should* spend time with you. The same is true for nurses, physical therapists, and any other ancillary healthcare professionals. *It is their job to take care of you.* Just as in any profession, some will be better at it than others. Find the ones that make you feel comfortable, give you the time you need, validate your concerns, and come up with smart strategies.
- **Give your team collaborative feedback.** Maybe you're working with the top specialist in your disease, but they don't have the best bedside manner. In that case, take a pause, put on your grown-up pants, and be bold with your feedback. Say something like, "I appreciate

that you are the best doctor in this area, and I'm very happy I'm in your care. But I need to communicate with you differently, because I sometimes feel like you don't have time for me. Are you open to that discussion?" As long as you do it from a place that's collaborative (ahem, *not* like I did early on, where I yelled profanities at the asshole), they will stop and get the wake-up call. And if they don't—well, that may be a deal breaker. And you're allowed to make that call.

Remember: take in as much information as you can handle and lean on the community around you for help. Take this one step at a time—or, if you've lost the use of your legs, like I did—one rotation of the wheels at a time.

PATIENT PERSPECTIVE: CHRISTY D., RELAPSING MS

Words can't describe how I felt the moment I heard the words, "You have MS." I was thirty-six and engaged to my soulmate; my career was advancing; my future was bright. I had done all the right things: I ate right; I exercised; I watched my weight; I didn't smoke; I didn't drink (well, not too much). But in an instant, my future went dark.

Words like "incurable," "disability," "progressive," and "unpredictable" consumed my thoughts and I felt alone. There were many challenges, both physical and emotional. I tried to move forward and embrace life with MS. But it was depression, not life, that embraced me in return and left me feeling alone and without hope. That was twenty-three years ago.

My life today is much different. I'm married to my soulmate. My work is challenging yet incredibly rewarding. I have wonderful family and friends. My days are full and rich. So, what happened? Someone reached out and shared her journey of living with MS with me. Then she invited me to reach out and share my journey with others. And I realized that I was not alone. I was *not* without hope. Through connecting with others, I realized that my life was not defined by a diagnosis, but by the choices I make every day. I am forever grateful that someone made the choice to reach out to me. And now, I choose to reach out to others.

YOU ARE NOT YOUR DISEASE

The identity earthquake that comes with a diagnosis is normal. As awful—or perhaps as encouraging—as that sounds, this is a *temporary* normal.

Temporary—that's the key point. If you can move down this Patient's Journey, get the right treatment, put together the right team of healthcare professionals, surround yourself with a support team of family and friends, and navigate the identity earthquake, *you will come out on the other side being you again.*

And you will be you, whether or not you can walk. You will be you, even if you physically look different. You will come back to finding the essence of who you are. I can promise you, because I've seen the journey unfold in literally tens of thousands of patients.

You will come out on the other side being you again.

It's going to take some time. Don't beat yourself up about that. The sooner you can accept your temporary new normal, the quicker you can get back to finding who you've always been. The faster you'll integrate your diagnosis into a new, fuller sense of self.

STAGE 2 OF THE PATIENT'S JOURNEY: DIAGNOSIS

- *Common emotions: relief, fear, a feeling of unreality, shaken identity.*
- *Common pitfalls: not asking for needed help, equating your identity with your disease.*
- *Your best next step: Strengthen your connections to others to get the help and support you need. Strengthen your own self-connection to fortify your sense of identity.*

CHAPTER 4

Grief

LAYERS OF LOSS; THEN, HOPE

"Hopelessness overtakes us when we are all alone, spinning hellish scenarios in our minds about which we cannot do anything. After all, how can we change something that doesn't really exist? But when we focus on reality, we almost always discover that there is something we can actually do to improve every situation. Every person has some power, and exercising our agency gives us hope."

— *Yuval Noah Harari*

It's grief that follows swift and hard after the diagnosis. In the Grief stage, everything feels awful.

But your story doesn't end here. The best way to get through this phase of the Patient's Journey is to make choices that reflect *hope* in your future and lead you to a better outcome.

I love the quote by author Yuval Noah Harari that I opened this chapter with: " … Every person has some power, and exercising our agency gives us hope." That's how I want you to understand "hope" in this chapter. Hope is not wishing and dreaming. Hope is *action*—a deliberate choice to exercise the agency you still have. And here's why this kind of hope matters so much: the Grief phase is heavy and exhausting. Grief is inevitable, and it is appropriate and necessary to allow it to wash over you. The fastest way to get through this stage is not to fight it or try to stuff it down, but simply to allow it to hit.

That's not easy—you may at times feel like you're drowning. But hope will be your life preserver.

And I do mean that literally.

"YOU MAY NEVER WALK AGAIN."

" ... This is confirming, along with your clinical examination, the diagnosis of multiple sclerosis."

When I heard my doctor say those words, I said, "Are you kidding me?"

She shook her head. "No."

"Am I going to be disabled for the rest of my life?" I asked, feeling panic rising. "Am I going to be able to walk again?" All the reading I had done about MS to that point had referred to it as "the crippler of young adults." *Don't let that be my story. Don't let me be young and crippled.*

My doctor took a breath. "Your type of multiple sclerosis is likely relapsing-remitting. There are currently no treatments available to address this, other than symptom management. Historically, the natural progression of patients with multiple sclerosis is that they are either ambulatory dependent, meaning they need an assistive device, like a walker or cane ... " She hesitated. "Or they are no longer ambulatory at all within ten to twelve years."

"You mean, in ten to twelve years, I could be permanently stuck in a wheelchair? In ten to twelve years, I won't ever be able to walk again?"

She held my gaze. "In ten to twelve years, you may no longer be able to walk."

I began crying my head off. I kept saying, "What is this going to mean for my life? How am I going to take care of my daughter? What am I going to do?" Thinking of the implications of my disease made me feel completely emotionally paralyzed—just like my legs. "Let's not get ahead of ourselves," my doctor said, trying to reassure me. "Some patients have a big attack. *You* are in the midst of a big attack. Sometimes an attack lasts a short period of time; sometimes it lasts a long period of time. We're working to fight your current attack by putting you on IV steroids to decrease the inflammation in your body. Tomorrow, we're going to start physical therapy and occupational therapy, and we're going to do everything possible to help you." She paused, waiting for my panicked breathing to slow down. "Your MS goes in waves, a relapsing and remitting cycle. There are attacks, then those are often followed by a period of quietness, usually still with some sort of neurological deficit. We're going to try to fight this attack. And then, we'll see what baseline you get back to."

Much of what she said washed over me completely. I was too overwhelmed to process it, fixating on the "fact" that I was going to be disabled for the rest of my life, paralyzed from the waist down before turning forty. It was like a ton of bricks falling on me, or being swallowed up in an earthquake.

But in the long hours that followed, my mind found its way back to one word: *baseline.*

If there was anything positive about that conversation, it was that nugget: the concept of a baseline. *The attack could quiet down. I could get back to a baseline.*

And if my baseline turned out to be better than this—then maybe I *could* walk again. I didn't have the progressive form of MS.

I had a relapsing-remitting form of MS, and that became my laser focus. That's what I decided I had to hang my hat on. *Gotta get back to baseline.*

Unfortunately, neither my body nor my emotions seemed to want to cooperate with my will. Both felt equally stuck. And most of my hospital visitors seemed to make things worse. I was in the hospital for about ten days, and during every one of those ten days, I felt subjected to a revolving door of sympathies. While I appreciated the concern when I reflected on it later, at the time, it felt more like people were stopping by to look at the monkey in the zoo.

It wasn't just the gawking that was problematic. The IV steroids being pumped into my veins caused me to become immunocompromised. And one of the well-wishers visiting the zoo brought a virus, not a banana.

On Christmas Eve, I was discharged. The plan was to enjoy Christmas with my family and continue my therapy with specialists who would visit me at home. But that plan went to hell when a minor cold I'd caught from a hospital visitor blew up into pneumonia and I had to be readmitted to the hospital. The MS attack that had just been "calmed down" was back in full force.

I rang in the New Year in the hospital: hooked up to an IV, getting pumped full of medications to cure the infection in my lungs and the worsening MS attack. After the infection passed, I was finally deemed stable enough to be sent home to recuperate, but only barely. My body was weak and the MS flare was still present. I could barely stay awake, I could not walk, my left arm was out of commission, and I was puffed up due to the steroids. And that was just on the outside.

On the inside, I was full of fear—scared to pieces, actually. I was sad and felt the first tight grip of grief, as tight as the MS banding symptoms had been around my midsection.

And the fun wasn't over yet. A few weeks later, I was given new medication to manage another symptom, and, unfortunately, we did not know I was highly allergic to it.

And unfortunately, I went into anaphylactic shock.

And unfortunately, I had a heart attack and nearly died on the floor of my home.

I was rushed back to the hospital—my blood pressure was thirty over fifteen. I remember this moment as though I was hovering over the bed. I heard the medical staffers calling for my dad. I saw my own body below me, saw the bells and lights going off, heard the nurses call for the crash cart, and saw people rushing around.

(Interestingly, I *didn't* see a heavenly light calling me to the great beyond. Apparently, God wasn't ready for me yet. Or else, the angels were like, "You say 'fuck' too much, Brenda, you're staying down there!")

So much for getting back to baseline.

Three days later, I woke up in the ICU. I had to stay there for another week to stabilize. After that, I was still too sick to go home, so I was transferred to an inpatient neurological rehabilitation ward.

I thought I had hit bottom in the days leading up to my diagnosis, but in this incredibly depressing place, I found a new low. Nobody was like me. There were no young people with MS. All my fellow patients were at the end of their lives with neurological conditions like Alzheimer's and severe Parkinson's. It was the last stop for a lot of these folks.

I had to press a button every time I needed someone to put a bed pan underneath me to pee or poop. The IV steroids were blowing all my veins and the nurses started inserting needles in my neck and feet. I saw zero progress—not in my body, not in the therapy tests I kept failing, and most of all, not in my emotions.

It was one of the most depressing places I've ever been. It felt like prison. I was overwhelmed by feelings of hopelessness.

Every day, my dad picked up Stephanie from school and brought her by to visit me. I'd try to put on a cheerful face and ask her about her day. I still can't even imagine how hard it must have been for her. As they prepared to leave, my eyes welled up. I knew the hell I'd return to as soon as they left.

"Stay positive, Bren," my dad would urge gently.

But how?

THE HEAVY REALITY OF GRIEF

I'm going to talk a lot about hope-inspired action in this chapter. We're going to talk through specific steps you can take to cultivate a mindset that *chooses hope*, one that works toward a better "baseline" than where you're at now. In those darkest of days for me when I was on the inpatient neuro rehab floor, it was hope that finally triggered a major shift in my mentality. The grief of dealing with my MS was still ever present, but eventually, there was something else. There was *hope* that it might not always be this bad. There was *hope* for better days around the corner. Hope changed everything.

However, before hope and renewed energy enter the Patient's Journey—either mine, yours, or anyone else's—grief hits. And the only way to move forward is to look that grief square in the face.

In my life, grief carved out a chasm between Brenda-Before-MS and Brenda-After-MS. I experienced a loss in my abilities; and for my family members and my daughter, the hopes and dreams we all had for my life suddenly seemed to evaporate. And for a while, that grief was appropriate to engage. It showed me that my illness was real.

The Grief stage is miserable, but it's also really important. It's appropriate, given the loss you've sustained. It also signals you've successfully moved out of the denial that can characterize the first two stages.

One of the titles I considered for this book was *The Patient Patient*. That's because you have to be damn patient while on this Patient's Journey. There are many stages of the Journey, and at every stage, there are stages *within* the stage. That's especially true for grief. Grief is not a one-and-done experience. It comes in different shades and colors, with different levels of intensity, with different durations. The acute stages of grief come first, and then follows a heavier, duller sense of loss. But every variation of grief is going to want to have its dance with you.

Grief comes in different shades and colors, with different levels of intensity, with different durations. Acute grief is eventually followed by a heavier, duller sense of loss.

Relief Grief

When my doctor said the words, "You have multiple sclerosis," I felt grief, but it wasn't like the grief I experienced four months later.

It was like a *relief* grief. On the one hand, there was tremendous sadness to know I had a chronic, debilitating condition. But on the other hand, I also felt relieved to know I wasn't making it up. If there was a label attached to me, I thought I could start doing something about it.

Anyone who has managed to get themselves a name for what's happening to their bodies should take a moment to register this relief. There are many people who live with debilitating symptoms that *don't* have a name, and they endure the constant fear of the unknown. They can't get away from the question, "What's wrong with me?" And that's incredibly hard. You can't even start the grief process because you don't know what the hell you have. You just know that your life and your family's life is blowing up in front of you.

If and when you get a name for what's going on—that's a milestone. It's awful to have something so scary confirmed, but it's also a weight off. *There's a name for it.* My doctor's hand was on my shoulder after she said that, and I took a deep breath. She moved her hand, and I dropped my shoulders. It was a moment of resignation: "Okay."

The initial grief that comes with a diagnosis is often coupled with relief to finally have a name for what you're dealing with.

Comprehension Grief

The next form of grief begins with a question: "So ... what is this shit?" I had a general knowledge of what multiple sclerosis was, but

I didn't really know the impact it would have on my life. There was a new level of grief that came as I began to comprehend the full magnitude of my neurological condition. The social worker would come by with a pamphlet, or someone would drop off a library book, or someone would stop by for coffee and share a story about their crippled auntie that died of complications related to MS. You wouldn't believe how many stories I heard about people "dying from MS"—even though modern research shows that it's very rare to die from MS. As my comprehension expanded about what this disease might entail, all of that *sucked*.

New knowledge about the challenges and risks that faced me with this disease led to intense grief. That was the sobbing and shaking under the covers stage. And for me, it was probably the most brutal. I still have sadness at times, over thirty years later.

New knowledge about the challenges and risks that face you with this disease can lead to intense grief.

Future Fears Grief

Comprehension grief slides right into future fears grief: all the "what ifs" As you learn about all the things that *could* happen to people with your condition, you naturally start to wonder what *will* happen. And without meaning to, you start to burden yourself with a lot of grief about things that may never come to pass.

For instance, when I thought about my future, I grieved never walking again. I grieved my early death. I grieved never going back to work, never driving again, never falling in love again. I grieved about my daughter becoming a social outcast because her mother was in a wheelchair. I grieved my bankruptcy.

None of those things ever happened. But the fear of them happening felt very real.

On certain days, it may help to remind yourself that "borrowing trouble" from tomorrow is useless, and that you're much better off just focusing on today. But other times, this "future fears grief" is just overwhelming. In fact, it's easy for me to go back to this place, even now. My MS can always suck me back down. I could still lose my ability to walk or see, so this grief—to some extent—lingers in your peripheral vision. There are always new future fears you can generate. How you learn to deal and cope with them is a lifelong skill you're going to need.

Future fears grief revolves around the "what ifs" of your future—but often, this is unnecessary stress. Many of these fears will never happen.

Empathy Grief

Another weird form of grief that came early on was the weight of trying to be strong for other people. I didn't want people feeling sorry for me, so I felt a self-imposed pressure to not let them see how torn up I was. With one or two exceptions, I tried to keep it together in front of friends and extended family members. I knew if they saw what a complete hot mess I was—how truly sad and stressed—they would worry even more about me.

I didn't want them to worry more, partly for them, but partly for my own self-preservation. I didn't want the onslaught of that added shit every day: the questions—"Are you okay? What does this mean? How are you *really doing*?"—the tears, the heavy sighs. I found people around me needing reassurance, but I didn't have the emotional capacity at that point to reassure everybody else. I could barely deal with my own grief!

My strategy was to try to mask it most of the time—which most psychologists would probably say is not the healthiest of strategies. But it was the coping mechanism that felt most available to me at the time. You'll need to identify your own best strategy to ride out the empathy grief. The strategies I shared to strengthen your own self-connection will help. I just knew that when I tried to share my intense grief with others, at that point in time, it elicited responses that I couldn't deal with.

Empathy grief describes the weight of trying to be strong for other people when you're barely hanging on yourself.

Reentry Grief

For any patients that spend a certain amount of time at an inpatient facility, there's a reentry point when you return home. You think that's going to be the happiest day of your life; and on the one hand, it is. But there's another form of grief that coincides with it. I was hit hard with this grief when I was finally released from the neurological rehab ward in May and moved back home.

I had walked out of my house on my own two legs—granted, one was being half dragged, but I was upright. Yet when I returned home, I was in a wheelchair. I couldn't do anything I remembered being able to do. I had been craving familiarity, but nothing was like the last time I was there.

That's the heartache of reentry grief: you arrive home, but nothing feels the same, because *you* aren't the same. When you come into that entryway and take everything in, your illness highlights new losses. You have to refamiliarize yourself with every part of your daily routine, getting around your house, and the activities of daily living. You have to learn new ways to accept and adapt to your changed set of circumstances. The familiarity of your surroundings can be a constant reminder of everything you've lost.

During reentry grief, the familiarity of your surroundings can be a constant reminder of everything you've lost.

These are the initial forms of grief: relief grief, comprehension grief, and grief related to future fears, empathy, and reentry. In my mind, they're the acute forms of grief.

When the intensity of that acute grief wears off, that's when you feel a quieter yet deeper sense of loss.

Loss

After dealing with a few forms of acute grief, you get to a place where you're capable of processing the changes to your life more thoughtfully. There's a bit more time for reflection, and a bit less intensity in your treatment. For me, that's when I had the time to process my grief as a loss. Although loss doesn't feel as paralyzing as acute grief, it also doesn't really go away, because you're feeling sad about things you've *lost* which you may never get back. This lengthier season of loss allows more space for reflection but still carries the weight of sadness.

And it felt like there was a *lot* of loss. There was a loss of my sense of self. I felt the loss of my independence. There was a loss of my potential—I knew I had a disease that, while it probably wouldn't kill me, would still alter the course of my life. I felt loss in my ability to parent my daughter the way I wanted to. There was no shortage of changes to mourn. It was incredibly sad to think of some of these things, but *I was processing*. And the very fact that I finally had the ability to *process* helped me start moving to other stages in my Patient's Journey. That will likely be true for you as well.

Acute grief eventually subsides, and you start coming to terms with what you've lost. This lengthier season of loss allows more space for reflection but still carries the weight of sadness. You can help yourself move forward in the Patient's Journey with intentional reflection.

Eventually, the noise of your acute crisis will settle down—when you've left the hospital, or you've had your first chemo infusion, or you've moved to the outpatient clinic, for example. Even then, the noise will follow you for a while; friends, neighbors, and community members knock on the door with their casseroles. Your family will probably be on pins and needles, wondering, "How is this going to go? Who do we need to get to look after her?" Appointments with different therapists and doctors will crowd your calendar.

But once all that stuff calms down, there's some space. And that's when it becomes much easier to process. That's when you have the mental space to consider, "Whoa—here we are. We're not in Kansas anymore."

It was in this stretch where I leaned into many of the strategies I recommended in the previous chapter: I did a lot of journaling. I did my cassette tapes with the recorded meditation. I did a lot of self-talk.

I needed that quiet space to accept the grief and internalize the fact that this had happened to me. In the quiet, I was able to spend time truly mourning the loss. And out of that processing and mourning and reflecting, I found the energy I needed to move forward.

MESSAGE TO CARE PARTNERS: YOUR GRIEF

As the care partner to a patient on this journey, you'll have to navigate your own layers of grief as well. In fact, you'll likely take your own full trip through the Patient's Journey, only you may travel it at different stages than your loved one. Be patient with each other as you find yourselves working through different stages and emotions at various times. By familiarizing yourselves with the stages, you'll both be able to show empathy for each other and can better meet the other person where they're at—wherever that may be. Suffice it to say, though, you *will* feel grief. But the way it manifests will be unique to you.

When I was in the early phases of my MS, my mom's grief seemed to be colored by feeling she had done something wrong—and this is common for mothers. She was asking herself, "What did I do wrong?" Of course, she had done nothing wrong, but in those days, I didn't have the emotional wherewithal to reassure her of that—I could barely hang on for myself. It was only many years later that I was able to reassure her with my words and actions that she didn't do anything wrong. But at times, I think she felt insecurity, guilt, and the grief of feeling like she must have *somehow* been responsible.

My dad experienced some of those same emotions, but he channeled his grief into looking for a way to *fix it*. It was hard for him to realize that he couldn't—there was no way for him to fix my MS. He had money to fix things, he had intelligence to make repairs—but he couldn't fix this. All he could do was drive me around, take care of errands, and do a few things around the house. That felt hugely insufficient for him.

That "fix it" response is true for many people: they want to find a way to make things unbroken. There's a nearly overwhelming grief that comes for some caregivers when they realize there's nothing you can do for this person you so desperately care for. For that reason, it's incredibly important for care partners to have somebody to talk to, *other* than the patient. You need a safe person to talk to and lean on because most of the time, early on, your sick person will not be able to provide you with the needed emotional support. I could not provide emotional support to *any* of the people in my life. The only person I could only marginally get there with was my daughter, and that was purely from the sheer force of a mother's love. I knew, if there was anything in me to give, it needed to go to her. But even then, I couldn't fully give her what she needed.

And yes—your kids will be coping with grief, too. There's good news and bad news when it comes to how children may cope with a parent's illness. On the one hand: children are extremely adaptable. Especially in the case of young children, they often don't know what they don't know. As a five-year-old, Stephanie got used to her mom being in a wheelchair and it was no big deal for her. We didn't try to magnify it, either. We chose to share appropriate information about my illness for where she was developmentally, which at that time was simply, "Mom's legs aren't working right now, so we're going to use this." Stephanie never acted out in school. There were no signs of trauma or stress coming out in her artwork. She did well in school and had lots of friends. In many ways, she seemed to roll with the changes pretty easily. But that doesn't mean it was easy or she wasn't affected.

The bad news is that kids will still experience their own grief. They can't be shielded entirely, and it's likely their grief will still manifest in either large or subtle ways. Some kids *may* act out at school or at home. Some children wet the bed, or quit activities they once loved, or show other signs that they're emotionally struggling. In the short term, Stephanie became more withdrawn—a little less open to new people and experiences. These signs often concern parents, but in one respect, their acting out is healthy: they're working to process and release their emotions. They're also alerting the adults in their orbit that they need emotional support.

There may be long term effects too, and that's not your fault—it's simply a reality. Stephanie told me recently that, for as long as she could remember, she felt she could lose her mom at any minute. Especially given that it was just her and me for most of her life—that's heavy. That was a significant burden for her to carry. She got used to taking care of me and looking after me, which also meant that when she became an adult, we had to sort through codependency issues. Much of that was born out of the ways she found to cope with her loss and grief at such a young age. And like my mom, I found myself asking, "What did I do wrong?" The answer remains the same: nothing. But this will affect you and the people you love.

The takeaway for care partners and other close family members or friends is that *you also need to process your grief.* Whether that's through journaling, meditation, seeing a counselor, talking with a friend, lining up a regular night out, indulging in a hobby, or going for regular walks—your own self-care and attention to your emotions is incredibly important. You are going through one of the hardest times of your *own* life, and you're carrying the burden of being one of your person's main supports. Care for yourself, so that you remain able to care for them.

It is crucial that care partners intentionally process their grief with a safe person, so they remain capable of offering support to their patient.

GIVE YOURSELF PERMISSION TO GRIEVE

For patients and care partners dealing with the grief of a weighty diagnosis, it's like all the pieces of your life suddenly feel shattered. That's the identity earthquake, right? In a cataclysmic event, everything falls apart.

Grief comes because it feels like we'll never have *that* life again. We want to reassemble all those broken pieces like we would reassemble a puzzle. We want to make the same exact picture. But as we start picking up some of the pieces, we realize that many of them are broken or bent. Some are lost altogether. Some are so broken you can't even tell what piece they belong to. In short: we're not getting that same picture back. That old life is gone—and that's why we feel such loss.

But that's not the end. I'm going to challenge you to embrace the mindset of an artist with all these broken pieces. A mosaic is made from shards of tile or glass, and every one of those shards used to belong to something else before they made a new picture. The difference between a puzzle and a mosaic is that the mosaic gets to be something brand new—something the artist decides on. There's no preordained picture printed on the cover of a box, telling you where each piece should go. *You* get to decide. The new image can be what you want it to be. You can choose how you arrange the colors, how you create the shapes; you can invent and define a new picture.

Take all the shattered pieces of your diagnosis and your pre-diagnosis life and put them together to make a new, colorful, rich mosaic for your life. Life doesn't stop with your diagnosis. It transforms. And it can transform into something beautiful.

Life doesn't stop with your diagnosis. It transforms. And it can transform into something beautiful.

Believe it or not, grief starts the process of this profound transformation. Grief is what enables you to acknowledge the pieces are broken and you're not going to be able to create the same picture you had before. It's painful. It's necessary. And it wakes you up to the fact that you *must* create something new.

You can't shortcut the Grief stage of the Patient's Journey. You can't Pollyanna your way out of it. Grief is often said to come in waves and sometimes it may wash over you at the most unexpected time, triggered by something small.

You must give yourself permission to *allow* that wave of grief to pass through you. If you do not give yourself permission to grieve, you will not progress in your Patient's Journey. I wish I could tell you that you would! But based on my own experience and talking to thousands of other patients—you will not. Grieving is a necessary experience on this journey.

And that's okay. It's normal and appropriate to grieve over the changes disease brings to your life, just as it's normal and appropriate to grieve the death of someone you love. Working through grief is what enables you to emerge on the other side as an emotionally healthy, intact person.

But when a loved one passes on, you don't want to *stay* in the place where you're feeling the same crushing grief as you felt on the day of their funeral in perpetuity. Eventually, you want to get to a place where you can remember the happy times with them: the good memories, the things they taught you, the experiences you shared.

The same is true for allowing yourself to eventually move on from the grief that comes with disease. However long it takes you, you will start to notice the acute grief and deep loss slowly give way to a kind of calmness. You will start to consider—*what's next?*

That's when it's valuable to start embracing new dreams for yourself. A dream isn't just something you have at night when you sleep. From your sick bed, or from your wheelchair, or from your chemo recliner—you start dreaming of a life less defined by illness. I remember dreaming that I would one day be able to make toast for Stephanie by myself again. I dreamed that I might beat the odds and one day be able to walk again.

It's choices—many repeated choices—that take your dreams out of the reverie of sleep to become the new contours of your life. Your dreams as a patient can become your reality. They can come to fruition if you have hope and follow your hope with action.

It's *hope* that drives choice.

THEN, CHOOSE HOPE

Hope is a game changer. Despair is immobilizing, but hope can inspire action. It can be the main motivating factor in choosing a positive next step.

Despair is immobilizing, but hope can inspire action. It can be the main motivating factor in choosing a positive next step.

After the chaos of moving home calmed down and I allowed myself to begin processing the loss I incurred due to MS, I found that I had the energy to ask myself some rhetorical questions. In my journal, I wrote things down, like: *Brenda—do you know that you can still plan your life? Do you know that you can still do things from a wheelchair?*

I gave myself the right to cry and experience the loss. That opened the door to a space where I could move *past* it and discover the choices I still had before me.

And I literally told myself, *You have a choice, Brenda*. It didn't initially feel like I had any control over my circumstances at all, but I finally recognized I *did* still have some agency.

It made me think of the game shows I grew up watching in the '70s, like "Let's Make a Deal." Those images came to mind as the stark alternative I faced: it was either Door 1 or Door 2. *Do you want to accept this grief and move past it? Or do you want to remain stuck in this sadness and bitterness forever?*

Then, I heard the little mantras my parents had raised me with. My mom—who happened to *be* on *Let's Make a Deal*—is the Queen of Fun. Her entire ethos as she raised me was to make life colorful and full of laughter. And my dad is all about, "Stay positive." I would hear their cheery voices in my head and imagine their pep talks: "You can't change these things, but you can change the way you react to this. Give yourself grace, knowing that you're going to slip up and not every day is going to be good. You can choose the way you're going to move forward."

My grief started to give way to a grim sense of humor. I'd tell my dad, "I'm going to choose to be positive, even though I'm embarrassed about how I look, and my self-esteem has taken a big hit." He'd cheer me on. I would look at myself in the mirror and say, "I'm still Stephanie's mother. And I'm going to go to the school recital in a wheelchair, and I'm going to let people push me." I tried to do deliberate things to reinforce that there would still be a life for me, and I paired my actions with these sorts of "announcements" to try to train my inner thoughts to get behind the idea.

I took the medicine. I engaged with the physical therapy. I researched other ways to help my body heal. These were the ways I put hope into action.

In my peripheral vision, I could see many of the other MS patients I had met in support groups. Many of them had opted to *not* take the medication. They had no hope that it would do anything for them. I had a completely different approach. I *was* hopeful that the drug could slow down my MS progression. And if it slowed down the MS progress, I had hope that I would not be using a wheelchair in ten years. I had hope I would be able to reenter the workplace. I had hope that I could drive a car again.

I was determined to not let people define me as irrelevant, or physically incapacitated, or mentally challenged. I was *not* a loser. I was *not* incapable.

I let hope feed my aspirations and I used choices to fuel my hope. I thought, *Well—if I'm hopeful for it, then I have to choose and try.*

That's what got me beyond grief: I chose. I tried. I did.

Let hope fuel your aspirations. Use choices to fuel your hope.

DEFINING HOPE

Don't tell my dad this, but I think of hope as being more complex than simply "staying positive." Staying positive is an outlook. It's an approach—a reframing strategy. I'm not knocking it; staying positive as an outlook is *incredibly* valuable, and it's something you are in control of.

Hope is something even more. On the one hand, it's aspirational—like, I remain hopeful that there will one day be a cure for MS. I have hope that the advent of MedTech will open new doors for curing neurodegenerative diseases. When I decided I was going to one day walk again, that was not a realistic idea at that point; it was purely aspirational. Hope, in that way, is a bucket of progress. It's the belief that, "It's going to get better before it gets worse."

But hope is also action oriented. One reason I've fought so hard to push the life sciences industry forward and be a change agent in this field is *because* I've hoped for a cure for MS. I showed up to all those therapy appointments and gave it my all *because* I hoped my symptoms would regress. And this is where the positivity mantra helps grease the wheels: an outlook of positivity makes each hope-oriented action a little easier. They're symbiotic in that way. A kernel of hope in a better future drives an attitude of positivity, which in turn drives positive choices toward an even wider horizon of hope.

Hope is aspirational, and it's also action oriented.

DITCH THE VICTIM MENTALITY

What hinders hope? Two words:

"Why me?"

Let's talk about this inner "victim" narrative and why it's so important to fight—for both patients and caregivers.

By now in this chapter, I've acknowledged the weight and heft of the grief you're experiencing. This illness is no small thing. It's a life-changing, earth-shattering thing. You *know* that I empathize. The grief and the struggle are real. I lived this. I get you.

With that in mind, I'm going to ask for your blessing to now shift the conversation toward some tough love truth.

Look: bad shit is going to happen to all of us, or happen to people we love. As hard as this is, it's normal. True, the magnitude of what is happening to you or your loved one might be more extreme than what is happening to other families. It is totally normal, especially early on, to feel like the victim and ask those questions: "Why me? What did I do to deserve this?"

It's also normal for care partners to say, "I didn't sign up for this. I can't believe this is happening to my family. What the hell does this mean for me? And oh my gosh, I feel guilty for even thinking that, because my sick person has it even worse—but I still feel that way."

The shit is normal. The pain is normal. The "Why me?" is normal. And the guilt is normal. It's all *normal*. We're human beings. And it's very, very easy to get caught in the wallowing.

But here's what happens when you let yourself get stuck there: you go into a "no hope" zone. You put yourself in a "no choice" zone. I cannot give you a single example of a good story about someone that stayed in the "victim" mentality, for either a patient or care partner. There is not one good story of someone who maintained the attitude, "I got ripped off by life," yet saw their life go on to become something great.

There is not one good story of someone who maintained the attitude, "I got ripped off by life," yet saw their life go on to become something great.

Maybe there is one out there, but I've worked with thousands of patients, and I can't think of one. That fact alone should be enough to encourage you to let the victim bullshit go.

Life is not fair. The "fair" comes to town once a year, as my dear friend and business partner Corbin always says. You didn't do anything wrong. Nobody did anything to deserve this. Let that go.

I believe that *how* you choose to let this go and start moving forward is what truly defines your character. It's those choices that will determine what you're made of and what you become.

WHY HOPE IS A GAME CHANGER

In my lowest low, as I laid in bed thinking, "This is it. My life is over," I was void of hope. I was void of everything—I was a void slug. It was like, "Well, this is my life now: this bed, this computer, this view. This is it. I can't imagine anything else. I can't do anything else. I just can't."

Without hope, you lose the spark that starts your engine. That's why, for Snow Companies, hope is *such* a central focus of what we try to inspire in people. I like to think of us as "hope engineers." Because when we help patients get connected to their stories, discover the purpose and hope within them, then share their wisdom, it gives *other* people hope. And then, the hope compounds exponentially!

Hope is a game changer. Despair gets you stuck, but hope can get you to *move*. It drives progress and choice. Hope helps you construct a "can do" life.

This is true, *even if your diagnosis is terminal.* I have spoken with many patients who were given a fatal diagnosis and told the end was months or even weeks away. In those cases, the hope is not in longevity—as tragic and sad as that may be. The hope in those cases is that the choices you make right now until the end of your life will define your last moments, on *your terms.* Your hope is defined by the choices you make about the kinds of conversations you have with your loved ones. Your hope is to end well; to leave a legacy of a life well lived, unto your final moments.

I know of a woman who felt hopeful and happy about the funeral she designed for herself. That may sound morbid, but she exercised choice over every element of it. She planned to have hip hop dancers, and a choir—it was going to be a party. And she was happy that she'd been able to make all those choices herself and hadn't left it up to the interpretation of other people. I see tremendous courage in that. She held onto her agency and made positive choices to make every one of her final moments count. To the patients that have a terminal outcome: there are still many things you can exercise choice over, which can be defined on your terms.

And—at the risk of giving false hope—I'm going to also say it's not over until it's over. I've heard many stories where everybody had given up hope over a patient's recovery, and then healing happened that could only be described as a miracle.

Hope keeps you looking for opportunities to make moments count—to make subtle changes toward what is positive and meaningful.

STRATEGIES TO CHOOSE POSITIVITY

So, how do you blow on the spark of hope to make it burn a little brighter? How do you actively cultivate a mindset that will start to move you beyond the Grief stage? Here are some practical recommendations.

Get the Skill of Mental Fortitude

Both patients and care partners need to get the skill of mental fortitude. Pardon my French, but you've got to make this your fucking superpower. Because if you don't get a hold of your thoughts, you'll easily slide into the "no hope, no choice" category. Train your thoughts toward a hopeful narrative. Remind yourself that every day you get through makes you that much more resilient. It's the small, subtle choices that will truly define what you're made of.

Reframe

Reframe, reframe, reframe. This is a mental fortitude strategy, and I had to employ it constantly in the early days after my diagnosis. The minute I had a limiting thought, like, "Well, I can't do this because I have MS ... I'm going to look stupid ... I feel insecure about this ... I'm going to hold people back"—the *minute* I caught myself doing that, I would stop and force myself to reframe. (Mental fortitude!) I'd give myself a pep talk: "Wait a second. Who cares what other people are going to think about me? I would like to go outside and get some fresh air. And it will be good for me. And if I look strange, who the hell cares?"

I tried to reframe every less-than-positive roadblock that came into my head. I would self-check, then remind myself, "There's another way to look at this. So, what is it?" It took practice and discipline to get my brain to go there, but it was a major step in training my mind to think positively. Now that I'm older, I laugh that I worried about this so much!

There's another way to look at this. So, what is it?

Remember the People Who Love You

When I was a void slug of despair in bed, I couldn't make a move for myself.

But I sat up in bed for Stephanie.

It was because of Stephanie that I said, "I'm going to try one more doctor. I'm not giving up yet." And it was thanks to the help of my family that I made any progress with doctors or therapeutics.

Remember the people who love you. Even if you can't choose hope for yourself, let your love for people around you pull you out of bed and motivate you to keep trying.

And do me a favor: include yourself in that category. At Snow Companies, we lead an exercise with our patients where they write a letter to themselves. We ask them, "If you were to write a letter to your newly diagnosed self, what would the person you are today say to the person you were then?" I love reading these. The letters are filled with emotion and encouragement. A huge focus for all of them is about remembering *their why.* They describe *why* it is important to stay hopeful, to stay connected, to stay engaged, to stay positive. And when they read their own letters, patients are typically shocked to see their own progress.

Then, after writing the letters and seeing what concepts especially float to the top, they are given an index card on which to write one word. When we put all those index cards together, it becomes a Vision Board for hope. We take a picture of it and send it out to all of them, and it becomes a powerful visual tool. After they leave our retreat, and life resumes, and they get back to their day-to-day activities, they are able to come back to that image, like their own positivity manifesto.

This is why it matters. *This* is why we keep trying. *These* are the reasons to choose positivity.

I encourage you to think about the people you love; think about the *why* behind your motivation to choose hope. Then, keep that visual present. When there are dark or heavy times—when that grief descends once again—you can return to that image and remind yourself: "Oh yeah. *That's* why."

Get a Safe Person to Talk To

This is crucial for both patients and care partners: you've got to have a trusted person that can listen to you without judgment. Ideally, it's someone outside of your relationship, because you're each already carrying a lot.

This should be a person whose opinions and solutions you value at a premium, who will keep your word vomit safe and confidential. You need a safe place where you can say anything you feel and truly know you're not burdening the other person with whatever you're dumping on them.

Half of the time, this safe person will be a professional therapist, and that's completely legitimate. Half of the time, you may have that gift of a person in your life already. Pull them in close. You're going to need to lean on them for a while.

Don't Ignore Signs of Declining Mental Health

It's normal to have ups and downs; as I said, grief comes in waves. But if you notice emotional heaviness that goes beyond that—something that causes a significant change in your activities of daily living—that should be a cue to talk to a healthcare professional. For example, if you notice that you used to have energy to engage with people but you're now starting to withdraw and be more solitary—that's a red flag. If you have sleep disruptions that seem like they may be caused by anxiety or stress, that's another red flag. These are all things to discuss with your healthcare provider. And certainly, if you've started entertaining thoughts of self-harm, seek medical help immediately.

Dealing with illness is a significant, life-altering event, and many people do experience mental health struggles that need greater attention than a change in mindset. If you find yourself there, don't wait to raise your hand for help.

Take Care of Yourself

This should be obvious, but it needs repeating: Take care of yourself. Prioritize sleep. Take care of your nutrition. Don't put any more stress on your body than what it's already dealing with.

I'm not going to be a hypocrite; I've done it both ways. Although I live an improved lifestyle now and prioritize my mental and physical health, there have been other times in my life when I burned the candle at both ends. It did me no favors. Usually, it caused MS flare-ups.

We're all going to die of something, but the irony is many chronic medical conditions are *not* what you end up dying from—it's all the other comorbidities that go along with them. We have a plethora of cutting-edge information today about our health and the impact of lifestyle factors on longevity. So, pay attention. *Apply it.* Help your body along by giving it what it needs in terms of food, exercise, rest, and positive living.

Help your body along by giving it what it needs in terms of food, rest, and positive living.

Fake It till You Make It: Positivity When You Need It

When all else fails, if you're struggling to choose positivity, pretend you're operating with the brain of someone else. If you're really deep in that hole, attempt a little role-play. Think: "What choice would I make if I was a more optimistic person?"

Even if you're not feeling hopeful, or are struggling to make the connection between hope and choice, just ask yourself this question: Why should I give up on me?

Here's the answer: you should *not*. Never, ever, ever, ever.

Nobody's going to care about you like *you* care about you. I try to instill that truth in patients because *it's up to you* to care for yourself. And until you are the number one priority, it's going to be hard for your healing trajectory to fall into place. It's not selfish to care about yourself: it's the most practical thing you can do to enable you to care for the other people you love.

PATIENT PERSPECTIVE: STEPHANIE B., MS

Grief and MS are like twins in your family. They join your party ill-mannered—unpredictable, unexpected. They are best friends with anxiety, anger, and guilt. I have struggled all of my life to understand why they will not leave.

Thirty-one years ago, I personally experienced a huge paradigm shift concerning multiple sclerosis. At that time, there was a dearth of information about MS and very little help available to patients. I was devastated by the fact that there was no cure and felt completely overwhelmed by grief.

In the years since then, so much has changed. So much has improved for the better. But there are still two essential things that have not changed in all those years: 1) there is still no cure for MS, and 2) the grief that occurs living with this lifelong disease comes back in waves throughout one's lifetime.

After all these years, it is evident that I somehow found a way to manage a life with those twins, and that's been helped by the fact that almost everything has improved: MS specialists, disease-modifying therapies, societies, patient communities, social media. Still, sometimes the twins come, and they stay. Sometimes they forget about me. When they leave me alone, I focus and breathe. I soak up sunshine. When they come back, I tolerate them. Again, and again.

WHAT'S NEXT FOR ME?

Once I got to a slightly more stable place with my MS, I started sharing my story. At first, I just shared it with small support groups. But I've shared it many times a year since then, sometimes to audiences with thousands of people. I've been sharing this story for over thirty years.

And consistently, when I describe the Diagnosis phase and the grief that followed, I still weep.

The grief is real. And in some ways, those various shades of grief will be ever present. But there's a way the grief becomes a part of you, rather than all of you. And accepting it deepens your capacity for compassion and love.

Grief is normal. It's cyclical. It hurts.

But I'm telling you: this will pass.

My decision to choose hope and positivity in the midst of grief was not possible because I'm somehow special, or mentally strong. I didn't think I was made of anything that great. I was a void slug in bed. I was cussing out my doctors.

Yet, over thirty years later—after getting through all that I've been through, after forcing myself to develop the superpower of mental fortitude—I feel like there's nothing I can't fucking do. At the start of my Patient's Journey, I would have never, ever had the self-confidence to say that. The transformation came because I had to discover skills I didn't even know I had. I learned how to train my inner narrative. I learned to choose what was good, even when I felt lower than low. I learned how to be present and mindful about the skills I was honing, and how to implement them.

And because I did all that, I became more and more proud of who I was—not *in spite* of my MS, but *because* I had MS. My journey with MS had made me even cooler! I was even better. I was even *stronger.* And why? Because I never would have had to learn or implement all those new skills otherwise.

Ask yourself: "What's next for me?" You can remain in the paralyzing place of victimhood. Or, you can recognize the agency you still have to choose hope. It's either A or B; Door 1 or Door 2. In my mind, the right choice is pretty clear.

Recognize the agency you still have to choose hope.

Choose hope. Then, begin architecting your next step. On the other side of this, *there is something good.* You can hope for that.

STAGE 3 OF THE PATIENT'S JOURNEY: GRIEF

- *Common emotions: many shades of grief and loss.*

- *Common pitfalls: making choices that reflect pessimism in your future, i.e., failing to get needed treatment, not taking medications, etc.*
- *Your best next step: Choose a hopeful outlook and take actions that align with that aspiration. Cultivate a positive mindset.*

CHAPTER 5

Anger

USE THE ENERGY OF ANGER TO MOVE YOURSELF FORWARD

"It's hard to fight an enemy who has outposts in your head."

— *Sally Kempton*

As you process the intense sadness during the Grief stage, and all those *Why me?* thoughts creep in, what happens next is natural.

You start to get angry about it.

Anger is a first cousin to grief. Whereas grief is defined by a sense of sadness, anger takes sadness and twists it into something hard that you can hit things with. Anger possesses more energy than grief, actively seeking ways to take control—but anger can also be more destructive, both for you and for everyone in your orbit.

Anger possesses more energy than grief, actively seeking ways to take control—but anger can also be more destructive, both for you and for everyone in your orbit.

Keep in mind there is an ebb and flow with each stage on the Patient's Journey. This Journey is not purely linear. You might exit the Grief stage and move into Anger, then slip back into Grief on a different day, and fast forward to the wisdom in the Acceptance stage the following afternoon. Grief *does* come. Anger *does* come. Acceptance—we hope—*does* eventually arrive. But their sequence, order, and layering are not as neat and tidy as mile markers on a hike. These are more like characters who walk with you for a time and meet up with you again down the road.

The *energy* in the Anger stage is a gift for your forward momentum—but only if you harness it productively. Think of anger as a wild mustang. If you were to try to ride an unbroken, wild mustang, the horse might run in chaotic, frenzied paths and exhaust you both. The ride could easily hurt you and take you far away from your loved ones.

But if you can *harness* the energy of the Anger phase, you can propel your life forward. You can break the mustang, get a saddle on it, and ride it like a racehorse toward the place you choose.

The way to do that is by making the deliberate choice to tell yourself a story that rejects self-doubt, fear, and self-pity. When you wrangle anger into that productive inner narrative, Anger can give you a needed burst of speed toward resilience and strength.

How do I know the destructive power of Anger?

I'll tell you.

GO TO HELL, MAN IN THE YELLOW HAT

One day, during the soul-sucking months of my inpatient rehab facility stint, I saw him: the Asshole Doctor—the jerk physician who had concluded I was crazy and suggested I might jump off the Golden Gate bridge. Talk about a negative narrative.

It doesn't rain often in California, but it was pouring that day. He must have just arrived at the hospital to do his rounds, because he hadn't taken off his coat. It was a bright yellow rain slicker—something Paddington Bear would wear, or Curious George's ridiculous friend. He even had on this goofy yellow hat. I saw him walk past my room as he was making rounds.

My reaction to seeing him was immediate and explosive—an effect that was most certainly exaggerated by the steroids I was being pumped full of. "Hey!" I yelled out to him. "Come over here!"

He gestured to himself: Who? Me?

"Yes, YOU," I said loudly. "Don't you remember me?"

He glanced at the outside of my door, looking for a chart that would give him clues. "I'm sorry, I don't ... "

I helped him out. "I was your patient and you told me that I was fucking crazy. You said I didn't have MS. Well, guess what? Guess what I have?!" I motioned to myself with my one good arm. "MULTIPLE SCLEROSIS. I *told* you I wasn't fucking crazy!"

His eyes got wide, but I wasn't done. "And I'll tell you what—you're a fucking *asshole*. I'm sure you're confirming your 'crazy' diagnosis of me as I scream and yell at you. But rest assured, I'm just really *angry*. Because instead of trying to do any kind of real test to see if I had MS, you told my dad I should be committed."

He stared at me in disbelief. "Apparently, I made a mistake," he said.

"You DID make a mistake. In fact, you made several mistakes," I said. "I think you need to go back to medical school and take a class that teaches you how to talk to people about their diagnoses. Because you took every bit of hope away from me. So, *shame* on you," I railed at him.

He shrugged. "I'm sorry," he said, insincerely. He nodded, making his yellow hat bob back and forth on his head.

"Get out, please!" I said to him. The Asshole Man in the Yellow Hat left.

That was vindictive, I know. But I was pissed, and at that moment, I wanted him to feel as shitty as he had made me feel.

The Anger phase had taken over and I had fury to burn.

ANGER COMES NEXT

What do you have to be angry about along this Patient's Journey? Let me count the reasons.

You're angry because this disease is messing up your life. It's ruining your plans and your health. Why should you be the one to get a disease like this? Why the hell did *you* get screwed over? This is impacting your kids or your marriage or your parents or your friends. It's impacting your ability to be productive, make money, and contribute to society. That pisses you off.

You're mad at the healthcare system, too. The doctors don't give you enough time. None of the specialists seem to talk to each other. People don't call you back soon enough. You've got a stack of medical bills, and you can't afford to pay them. You're also mad at people who make stupid comments: people who try to be empathetic and end up insulting you. People who say they want to help and end up treating you like a helpless loser. No one understands. In this phase, everyone seems like an idiot.

You're angry at your own body because it's betraying you. The visible symptoms that people see erode your own self-esteem. Losing control of your bladder in a public space, an epileptic seizure, a fainting spell, dealing with the loss of all your hair—these are intensely personal, embarrassing experiences. You're angry at being humiliated over something beyond your control.

And you're angry that some people assume this disease *is* something within your control. You've had to take a lot of sick days and you know people are making assumptions: they think you're lazy, you don't do your job, you're not a team player. You're mad that some of your symptoms are *less* visible, because people don't even recognize that you're dealing with something that's a big deal.

But the people who know you're sick may annoy you, too. Some of those people have the audacity to treat you as though your IQ has dropped by 50 points. Why are people talking down to you all of a sudden?! As though you don't have the mental capacity to engage the way you did before your diagnosis. What are you, defunct? Damaged goods?

Or, if they don't treat you like you're stupid, they treat you with *obvious* discomfort. Clearly, they don't know what to say, or how to be, or what to ask about your *"condition,"* so they just trivialize and dumb down every conversation. There's no more substance to create a genuine human interaction. "I don't want to trigger you," someone says, WHICH IS SO DAMN TRIGGERING.

You beat yourself up over your own negative thoughts. Sometimes you internalize the negative messages: "I *am* a lazy patient. I am a public humiliation. People think I'm damaged goods. Who will ever love me? *I* wouldn't want to put up with me, so why would anyone else? My life is over."

Then you beat yourself up for beating yourself up. "Why am I staying stuck in such a bad headspace? Why can't I snap out of it? I'm such a loser. I hate myself."

You get sucked into an anger spiral about all the things you *perceive* your illness will do to your life. "I'm going to be alone. I'm never going to regain my strength. I'm going to be broke forever because of all my medical bills. My kid is going to be a social outcast because I'm a sick parent. I'm going to lose my cognitive abilities forever. I won't be able to travel ever again." I had every one of those thoughts, and not one of those fears became my reality. But it's hard to stop the momentum of anger—you pour energy and expend your emotions on things that may never even come to pass.

I remember this stage vividly. Early in my MS journey, the disease took away my ability to walk and be self-sufficient. I had always been very independent, and suddenly I needed to rely on other people—I didn't like that. I was angry at simple things: not being able to make toast, not being able to get my daughter to school. I was frustrated that a lot of the most mundane tasks in life—things I had always taken for granted—were now completely gone. I was pissed off at being sick and pissed off that there were people in the healthcare world that treated me like I was crazy—in fact, that still fries my ass, over thirty years later.

In the Anger stage, the grief that felt so deep and layered morphs into a dark, buzzing mass that makes you *angry at everything*. And this can lead to a dangerous, toxic narrative that can warp how you view the world.

Anger is understandable and normal. But, left unchecked, it can build a toxic narrative that warps how you view the world.

The Danger in the Anger Phase

Here's the danger in letting the Anger Horse run wild: you're going to isolate yourself, and it won't take long before that happens. If you stay in the place of victimhood and bitterness, you become unpleasant to be around. All of the help you desperately need is going to quickly be diverted because people won't want to be around you. If you're yelling or screaming at people, or treating others like shit, people are going to find something else to do. Nobody wants to be treated that way.

You also get the reputation of being a bad patient, which means you're going to see your healthcare partnerships suffer. You won't get time with the doctor. You won't get a call back. No one wants to deal with a belligerent, raging patient. And I'm not here to discuss the legality of that or the pros and cons of the healthcare system treating you badly. You're a paying customer after all—and you're entitled to be angry that all of this is happening to you. But setting that aside, it's a fact of human nature that people don't want to deal with someone who has a constant bad attitude, lacks civility, and spouts anger all the time. The nurses, doctors, and healthcare workers who you desperately need to be on your team will avoid you.

I speak from experience—as you may have gleaned from the story I opened this chapter with. (Not my finest moment.) And I've also observed how anger can lead to isolation in other patients. I've seen many marriages break up as a result of anger experienced by both patients and care partners. It's easy to forget the basic rules of civility when you feel so ill or so upset about the direction your life has taken. The words "please" and "thank you" stop coming out of your mouth at a time when your loved ones *especially* need to hear a basic acknowledgment of their efforts to help you. That can be damaging.

The anger has to go somewhere, so it often gets directed by spewing vitriol at other people. And if *that* happens, the anger will permeate your relationships—especially the most important ones. Anger can also burn your bridges with acquaintances. The lady from next door who shows up with her casserole doesn't want to be treated rudely. The other parents on the PTA don't want your sarcasm. These are the cold, hard facts: no one wants to be around somebody who's being mean to them, even if that person has a good reason to be angry.

Perhaps worst of all, anger can get you stuck in the hellish part of the Patient's Journey. Thankfully, I wasn't in the Anger stage for long, but I *was* there, and I've seen many people stay there. For the people who stay there, that's where they stop. The pity party becomes your reality. There's no more progress on the Patient's Journey; they remain in Anger.

Those patients who stay in a place of bitterness become chronic curmudgeons. They keep cycling between grief and anger, grief and anger. Rather than accept that this has happened to them, they just spin there and spiral down. Some days they're incredibly depressed. Other days, they're lashing out angrily. And as a result, they suffer needlessly. They keep themselves down with an attitude of victimhood, staying trapped in a constant blame game.

BUT—hear this great big "but"—there is a way to harness anger toward a more productive end.

In the early days after getting diagnosed with MS, I was not an engaged patient. I hated all the rehabilitation exercises they wanted me to do. I would tell doctors and nurses, "I don't even know why we're doing this physical therapy; I don't see that it's working. I'm never going to walk again." I had a bad attitude, and I projected that onto other people and blamed them for my lack of success: "The physical therapist is crappy. The neuropsychologist is a jerk." It was a constant blame game. But when I stopped putting so much energy into negativity, I had more energy to put into acceptance and a positive attitude. I was able to ask, "What can my life look like from this wheelchair?" That's when some of the tides started to turn for me.

What human on the planet—sick or not—doesn't like to see progress? When you put effort into something, you want to see progress. And when I became an engaged patient—*there was progress*. I was able to do things better than I could six months ago. And as I began to claim the power of a positive attitude, I regained a sense of control.

Everybody loves control. I *really* love control. When you accept your illness and recognize that some things are beyond your control, you open yourself to more effectively control the things that *are* within your power. You can harness your anger in a *competitive* direction. If you move yourself to a headspace where you've identified something to hope for or aspire to, then you can turn your progress into a competition with yourself. Instead of taking choices *off* the table for yourself, you can channel all that angry energy into doing the hard work to move forward: doing the therapies, taking the meds, scratching off another chemo infusion.

You've got to look to the other end of the tunnel. Otherwise, all of your personal growth and development as a person living with a medical condition will come to a hard stop.

Envision a story that includes a happy ending on the other side of this. Envision your true success. Envision yourself living with happiness and joy, despite illness. *That's* the productive end that anger can help you drive toward.

Envision yourself living with happiness and joy, despite illness. Use the energy from anger to help yourself drive toward that productive end.

THE GIFT IN THE ANGER PHASE: ENERGY!

In my own Patient's Journey, one of the things that served me the most was channeling my anger into action. I did that by harnessing my competitive spirit.

I'm incredibly competitive. If you put out Monopoly, I will beat your ass. If someone puts out Clue, I'm going to win. If I was playing Uno with a group of children, I would probably make them cry, because I would continue to beat them, hand after hand.

I'm not saying this is a good thing; I'm just saying it's how I'm wired.

And that competitiveness was *useful* to me. I thought of multiple sclerosis as a game I needed to win. *I needed to beat it*, and that's where I channeled my focus.

The silver lining of Anger is that there's some energy there. If you use anger to fuel your hope and choices, it can drive you to get out of bed every day and help you work toward healing.

I tell people that it's okay to get mad at their illness. It's okay to be mad at MS! It's okay to be mad at cancer! I love the tagline I see on bumper stickers and T-shirts: "Fuck cancer." That attitude is appropriate! And you can make anger work for you by showing that *you're absolutely better than your disease.* This is something to rage against.

I know some people who have given their anger a name, so they can more practically visualize it. One friend envisioned her anger as a giant pile of shit. Every time she thought about how angry she was at her disease, she imagined a giant pile of shit and it made her laugh. She told me, "I don't want that in my house!" Other patients I know have imagined anime-like characters, like an ugly robot or creature.

Go with whatever works for you—there are no rules to this journey. Everyone has to figure this out while they're in the midst of trying to move forward. But I've got a few more ideas to help you along.

Climb Out of the Anger Pit

Without a focus, it's easy to spin yourself out on anger and get mired in it. Here are some of the strategies I tried that actually helped me make forward progress:

- **Get up-to-date, accurate information.** I tried to generate to-do lists for myself that I could check off to help me feel like I was making progress. I made myself my own project plan. First and foremost, that meant building up my knowledge base. In 1993, when I got diagnosed, the information in the library about MS was from the fifties. My first project was to learn everything I could about the most up-to-date research around MS, so I would know the game I was playing. The more knowledge I had, the more I could move my chess pieces around on the board. That meant getting closer to putting MS in checkmate: boom. *I win.*

- **Connect with thought leaders who know your disease.** I wanted to talk to every thought leader on this subject, whether it was a healthcare professional, an ancillary expert in the field, or even another patient. Being able to connect with real humans who had expertise in my illness added to my knowledge while also providing opportunities to experience their compassion and understanding. That was a major morale boost.

- **Be fluid in your expectations.** At the same time, even as I was learning "the game" of my MS, plenty of things I tried didn't work. Some weeks felt like, "Go straight to jail. Do not pass GO, do not collect $200." But I had to accept those roadblocks as a delay, not as defeat. Setbacks with your disease can easily feel like they're beating you down. You're already tired, you don't feel well, you're still overwhelmed, and you're still battling grief—the setbacks can tempt you to give up hope. It's incredibly difficult in those moments to regroup and keep going. So, if you need a day, take a day. If you need a week or two, that's okay.

- **But then, keep going.** You *do* need to eventually get back up and try again. Hold yourself accountable to keep doing the work. There's no magical disease fairy that will help you snap out of this or miraculously deliver you to a better place. *You* have to do the work.

So, if you've taken a day, tell yourself, "Today's going to be an off day. I'm going to lie in bed. But tomorrow, unless there's something really physically wrong with me, I'm going to go at this a different way." Seek out the visual or concept that keeps you motivated. Find your reason to keep playing the game to beat the competition.

- **Tell yourself you don't have time to be angry.** Some cancer patients I've spoken with have told me a variation of this same theme: "There's no time to be angry. If I want to use the time I have left to be present, do good, and focus on the things that are worthwhile, I can't burn up my time being angry. I need to accept this disease and focus whatever energy I have on the things that are worthwhile in living life." I see a lot of wisdom in this. Anger is natural and appropriate—but if you let it spiral, it's not going to *get* you anywhere. Sitting in it ends up prolonging a really bad phase on this Patient's Journey.

In sum: finding energy in Anger means you're too stubborn to "let the disease have its way." It's about not giving up. It's about working hard to defeat the *real* enemy.

If you don't moderate your rage and get to a more constructive place, anger can easily be like "friendly fire": violence that ends up hurting your own potential for victory. The sooner you can let the outward anger go and direct that energy toward defeating the *disease*, the better off you'll be.

Ask yourself: What is the anger costing you?

It's probably costing you a lot. And it's not worth it.

That's why it's so important to harness the energy from your anger in ways that will help you. I've saved the most important strategy for last.

USE THE ENERGY TO SHAPE YOUR INNER NARRATIVE

Early on in the Patient's Journey, it's easy to tell yourself a negative, sad story. "I'm a loser. This only happens to bad people. Did my parents not take care of me? Did I offend karma in some epic way?" Your headspace is at risk of being taken over by a whole host of self-doubt and negative narratives—I alluded to some of them earlier in this chapter when describing all the reasons we feel angry.

After working for over thirty years to share my story all over the globe and inspire other patients to do the same, I've learned that it's profoundly healing to *take your narrative back*. Own your *own* personal truth. When you can be vulnerable about who you are and express that to other people, you find new power for yourself. And that power will be greater than the negative power you've been suffering from grief and anger.

PATIENT PERSPECTIVE:
JENN M., CARCINOID CANCER

When I was diagnosed with my terminal illness, my first instinct was to deny it and fight the changes that come with it. However, with all my energy going toward fighting, I realized I was giving it all my power. To take that power back, I had to allow myself to grieve my old life and stop fighting. I made the decision to embrace my new life, giving me the power to chart a new path.

Grief often brought self-pity. At times, I allowed myself to feel that. Whether that meant eating ice cream or bawling to a sad movie, I decided it was important to feel that rather than let it swallow me whole. However, I also realized it was just as important not to dwell in those feelings. After sitting on the couch with a Hallmark movie for a good cry, I would kick myself in the butt and get back to my new normal.

For me, that was focusing on the *can*, not the *can't*. I made up my mind to see life in terms of what I *can* do. I flipped the narrative so that when I hit a wall, I put the car in reverse and went in a different direction.

Looking at life with this perspective gave the power back to me, rather than to the disease. When I view life through the lens of "I can"—yes, even with a terminal illness—I see more open doors than closed ones. And I have the power to open even more, especially as I raise my daughters. I tell them, "When you focus on what you can do, you have the power of becoming your own advocate. You know what's best for you; you know what you can do. Live life as you see fit. Know your body, your goals, and how to achieve them. Don't let anything stand in your way."

There will always be voices out there who want to hold you down in negativity—both other people's voices and your own inner critic. "You're not this. You're not that." But if that's the audio tape you're playing on repeat in your head, that is what you become.

It's a simple fact of neuroscience that repetition rewires your brain. Much like when you train one particular muscle and let other muscles atrophy, repeating positive or negative thoughts will make that response more automatic. Point being: be careful what thoughts you think!

You have to be in charge of putting the good narrative about yourself out into the world. Start by putting it in your own head. *You* get to say what you can accomplish, how you're going to see the world, and how you're going to come to terms with this.

You have to be in charge of putting the good narrative about yourself out into the world. Start by putting it in your own head.

How do you claim your own positive narrative? You may think I'm crazy when I say what I'm about to say.

Paint yourself a picture of *what your disease is giving you*, rather than what it's taken away.

Don't throw the book against the wall. I know that's a big ask. But among the many thousands of patients I've spoken to, I cannot name a single person that hasn't acknowledged *there were eventual gifts* that came out of their experience with disease.

I've heard people talk about how they developed a perspective on what really matters, a deeper appreciation for humankind and their own lives. They are more grateful for their own stories and their own journeys. They talk about the *blessings* they've experienced as a result of their disease.

Disease will NOT feel that way early on. And, as I said in the previous chapter, some mental health challenges are severe enough that medication or professional help is needed, above and beyond your own mindset shift. Please, don't take this as me downplaying the gravity of the challenges you face in the Grief and Anger phases.

But I also don't want to downplay the incredible gifts that can come through this journey. Because I've heard countless stories from patients who were in complete despair or consumed by bitterness who *moved on* and found hope and transformation.

Incredible gifts can come through this journey.

When you can get there—when the world starts revealing itself with more shine and sparkle than it ever used to, because life feels that much more precious—that is something almost magical. That spectacular perspective makes everything else easier, and you only discover it on the other side of working through what it means to live with a disease.

That is true for me. I hope I've given you the smallest glimpse of the hell I endured early in my illness. But on the other side, there have been so many gifts. I am a better person post-MS, than I was pre-MS—a million times over. The changes happened while I navigated the long, complicated, emotionally messy journey that you yourself are on.

Develop a Thick Skin

Early on in my diagnosis, after I finally got out of the hospital (plot spoiler), I couldn't trust my legs for a long time. I was in and out of wheelchairs, and using walkers and canes for the first few years. But I still wanted to remain involved in my daughter's school, especially after I lost my job. I decided the silver lining would be that I could be much more present at Steph's school.

So, when a field trip was announced and they were recruiting parents to chaperone, I volunteered. I figured I could supervise kids from a wheelchair.

But the teacher called me. "We can't authorize you to go on the field trip as a volunteer," she said. Heavy sigh on the other end of the phone. "You just won't be able to keep up with the kids. It would be a liability to have you on the field trip. We're very sorry."

That was devastating. It hurt my feelings. It also fucking pissed me off. This teacher wanted to slap me with a narrative of incompetence, which was a narrative I was already fighting to unstick from myself.

Once I got done being devastated, my anger gave me a new idea. If I couldn't be the field trip mom, fine. I decided I was going to be the mom that went to the school *every day* to read books to the kids. I was going to be in that teacher's space as a permanent fucking fixture.

Once again, kind of competitive.

I called the school back. "I have a solution," I said. "No field trips." I gritted my teeth, still feeling pissed. "Instead, I'm going to read to the kids."

The voice on the other end made a polite, affirming noise.

"Every day," I said. "At least, every day I possibly can."

The voice on the other end made a slightly strangled sound.

I decided this was an opportunity to educate them. When I read to the kids in front of the teacher, I was teaching the *kids* about living with a disability, but it was even more so for the sake of the teacher. I wanted to make sure she understood that people with disabilities were no different than any able-bodied person.

On the days that I could, I showed up. I loved those kids. The teacher and I had several meaningful conversations about living with disease. By the end of the school year, she thought I was the greatest person she'd ever met in her entire life. I got some honorary "Parent of the Effing Year" award. *That's* the narrative I was going to own.

Listen: I want you to take the angry energy you're feeling in this stage and decide you're going to use it to come in hot and bold. People want to mess with your self-beliefs? Don't let them. People want to discriminate against you or treat you like you're unintelligent? Who the fuck cares? Look for opportunities to educate them otherwise. Don't try to hide your disease; put it out there and get accommodations. *You* take the lead in this conversation.

So much of this battle is fought through reframing. You have to reframe your own narrative for yourself, but you also have to teach others how to see you as a whole person. For years, I've introduced myself by saying, "I'm Brenda. I'm a wife, a mother, a businessperson, and I live really well with multiple sclerosis." I am many things. *You* are many things. You are not defined by your disease.

You have to reframe your own narrative for yourself, but you also have to teach others how to see you as a whole person.

I remember learning in a journalism class that, whenever you're writing a story, you always have to ask the *who, what, where, when, why,* and *how.* And I've found those prompts have been incredibly helpful when I want to reshape a bad narrative and turn it on its head. Here's an example.

Shitty narrative: "I'm sorry, but you can't go on the field trip."

Reframe:

- *Who* says I can't go on the field trip? The teacher. And the teacher was limited in her knowledge and understanding. The day she told me I couldn't go, I was humiliated. But later, I thought, "Hang on, is it even legal for her to say that?" The thought allowed me to question her narrative entirely and come to the helpful conclusion that she needed to be educated about a thing or two. Years later, I lobbied on Capitol Hill for people with disabilities. By thinking critically about the *who,* I was able to challenge the shitty narrative and take action that helped educate people about the underestimated capabilities of disabled people.
- *What* was the substance of what she was saying? I interpreted it as, "You're not like the other moms." That made me think, "Well then, I've got to figure out a way to show them that I *am* like the other moms."
- *Where* was this all taking place? It was a school thing, and in my case, the school was close enough that Stephanie could roll me there in my wheelchair. That enabled me to cheerfully and insistently insert myself into the teacher's classroom on the days that I could.
- *When, why,* and *how* all involved strategy. I intended to go every day—or, at least, as often as I possibly could, given my stamina. I was going to read to "the kids" to help educate the teacher about the capabilities

of people living with disabilities. (And, why not? The children, too.) And I was going to do it by reading books.

I'm now the founder and CEO of a company, but before I started any of that, I had to be CEO of myself. I was the CEO of my Patient's Journey. As a mom, as a daughter, and later as a wife—I had to operate in all those contexts as a CEO: deciding on and executing strategy, guiding a team, and troubleshooting problems.

This is how you take back your narrative. You reframe, you strategize, and then you get it *done*. Let your angry energy propel you along. The key to success in anything is to stop talking about it—whatever you want to do—and *do* it.

And if you don't have the energy yet to storm the gates of any negative naysayers, take a smaller step. Keeping a journal can be a powerful way to maintain a hold on your own narrative. Many meds affect your memory, as do stressful emotions. By keeping a journal, you can look back and audit what's working for you so you can replicate the helpful things. That will keep you moving steadily forward. I used to page through my own journal, being like, "What the hell did I do last time this happened … ?" And then I would find a journal entry and say, "Okay, yes—I'll do that again."

Whether you're telling other people your reframed narrative, or simply developing it for yourself, pick a good story. Shelve the narrative that paints you as a victim, or incompetent, or useless. Tell a story that includes all the possibilities that remain for you. Tell yourself a story of hope.

Claim a narrative for your life that includes all the possibilities that remain for you. Tell yourself a story of hope.

MESSAGE TO CARE PARTNERS: YOUR OWN THICK SKIN

In the Anger stage, patients may be venting a lot of anger and frustration—and unfortunately, that may often be directed at care partners. You, as the care partner, might even get inadvertently blamed for things that are not your fault. This isn't fair, but it's also common. As the cliché goes, "You hurt the person you love the most." Your loved one is hurting—and they may direct a lot of that hurt at you.

For this reason, the Anger stage is probably the hardest part of the Patient's Journey for care partners to weather. There may be blame, name calling, anger, frustration—90 percent of which is unfair and unjust. You've been giving, giving, giving—and this is the thanks you get?! And this, on top of your own grief, exhaustion, and anger at how your life is changed? The combination is brutal.

Many care partners will simply choose to bail. But for those who want to fight the good fight and stay in it, here's what you need to do:

- **Try not to be pissed at your person.** Their anger directed at you is not personal; they're angry at everything. You're simply their safest, most trusted person to vent the anger around. In that way, the rage vented in your direction could be considered a bizarre form of flattery. Do your best to develop thick skin and take it with a sense of humor. Be patient. This stage won't last forever (at least, if they keep reading this book, it won't); but while they're in it, they're going to have a hard time controlling themselves.

• **Give yourself permission to take breaks.** I've said this before to care partners, and I'll say it again: carve out space for yourself to live your own life. Breaks will allow your own emotions to cool and remind you that you're still an independent person. Breaks will also give you a chance to get some perspective on the pain your loved one is experiencing and help you return to your role as care partner with renewed empathy.

• **Schedule check-ins with each other during emotionally neutral moments.** There will be times when your loved one is in a state of accelerated anxiety or in the thick of dealing with medication side effects. That is not the time to discuss their expression of anger toward you. Instead, try to find a neutral time when you both feel calm and relatively good. Come to the table together. Acknowledge the spilled milk, then do your best to clean it up and reset. Gently and objectively share how you've felt about being targeted with anger. Give each other the chance to clarify intentions, emotions, and feelings toward each other. These moments will provide you both with opportunities to reflect and admit, "I never intended to lash out at you ... I'm just dealing with so much frustration, and fear, and grief ... " You both may have behavior to explain. Use these check-ins to ensure the accusations and bad feelings don't stick.

- **Learn to manage how you communicate.** Care partners will instinctively want to fix their loved one's problems, but if they only ever show up with cheery
solutions, patients will feel alone in their misery. The
resulting disconnect can be more counterproductive
than helpful and can easily prompt more anger and
verbal vomiting from the patient. So, do your best to
sense when your loved one needs something. Take the
emotional pulse of your conversations: Is now an
opportunity for you to just listen and not say a word?
Is it an opportunity to solve a problem? Is it an opportunity to say, "I want to validate how hard this is for
you. For the sake of all of our emotional health, let's
take a short pause. Let's regroup in thirty minutes."
When in doubt, simply ask your loved one what kind
of communication would be most helpful for them.

- **Remember that your relationship is not just "care partner and patient."** Relationships can atrophy if you lose
yourself in these new, hard identities. Remember who
you were as a duo before the diagnosis: lovers, spouses,
parent and child, best friends. Find ways to communicate on levels other than simply patient and caregiver.
And find things to do that help remind you of how
much you enjoy each other's company: watch a movie
together, drive somewhere with a view, or catch up
about life stuff that doesn't have to do with illness.

As important as it is for the patient to remember who they truly
are, you need to remember you're not "just" someone who waits

hand and foot on a sick person. And you *both* need to remember your relationship has far more depth, richness, and color than simply dealing with sickness together.

WEED THE GARDEN

If I had stayed angry, I would have compromised my choices and limited my ability to get well. Only because I ultimately *accepted* my illness and tried to construct a better life for myself was I able to start writing a new story with a better ending. If I hadn't moved to acceptance, there's a high probability that all of my worst fears about my future would have come to pass. But because I chose positivity—and because I employed the other strategies described in this book—I went on to have a better life with MS than I'd had before. In fact, if I had to choose between the two, I'd pick the life I've had *with* MS.

The most important thing you can do for yourself in the Anger phase is to define yourself on *your own* terms—don't let the anger define you. Don't let bitterness or resentment or anger take over your Patient's Journey. Channel the anger toward a productive end as best as you can, and ultimately, try to get rid of it entirely. I've had MS for over thirty years, and I've been mostly anger-free for about twenty-nine of them. (Don't get me wrong; I still have expletive-laden outbursts sometimes. But I no longer feel *trapped* in the anger pit.) I truly think one of the reasons I've had success in all aspects of my life is because I didn't let the anger fester or pollute who I was. I tried not to let it pollute my relationships. I'm not even sure I had the wherewithal to know that I was constantly looking for ways to get beyond my anger—I just didn't like how it felt.

As you try to care for your body and your mind in the midst of this sickness, think of it like tending a garden. Letting anger take root for any lengthy amount of time is like allowing a weed to grow in your perfect tomato garden. Left unchecked, it will ruin your potential for a good harvest.

Try to move through this stage as quickly as you can. Anger is normal, appropriate, and can even be useful if you harness the energy from anger to move you in a positive direction. But don't stay in the place of being pissed off and sorry for yourself long. Don't let anger become a weed in your soul.

Dig it up and move forward. The next stage is a major turning point.

STAGE 4 OF THE PATIENT'S JOURNEY: ANGER

- *Common emotions: anger, bitterness, a sense of victimhood.*
- *Common pitfalls: getting stuck in a negative mindset, disengaging from treatment, blaming people for your misery and establishing a reputation as a hard person to be around.*
- *Your best next step: Use the energy from anger to fuel your progress and healing; craft a positive inner narrative.*

CHAPTER 6

Acceptance

THE SECRET TO ACHIEVING GREATER CHOICE
AND CONTROL

"Acceptance doesn't mean resignation. It means understanding that something is what it is, and there's got to be a way through it."

— Michael J. Fox

For a long time, I viewed MS as the enemy. It was attacking me, and I had to fight it. When people talked to me about it, everything felt dark and negative.

That got old. And really depressing.

Things changed when I got to a point of acceptance. Accepting that MS was a part of me was a major mental reset. I had felt out of control for so long, but by setting aside anger and grief for acceptance, I realized there *were* some things in my life I still had control over. I still had choices. My life still held *possibility*.

That's the threshold we're going to cross in this chapter. The Grief and Anger stages contain a lot of heavy darkness, but Acceptance takes us around a corner where things get just a bit brighter. It's not an easy place to get to, but it's worth it. Acceptance may not be something you arrive at due to sheer will or positivity—it may be something you slump and fold into out of sheer exhaustion. But whether you leap over this threshold or drag yourself across it, life looks different on the other side. It's a little less violent. A little more calm. The battle sounds die down.

The months I spent in the neurological rehab ward were some of the lowest of my life. But I finally concluded that the ultimate decision maker of how I was going to fare was me. I could get the best medicine and the highest standard of care—but still, I knew all of that may or may not work. Even on my worst days, I knew that the only way forward was hope and positivity. That meant getting myself out of the war zone.

The only way forward is hope and positivity. That means getting yourself out of the war zone.

PUTTING HUMPTY DUMPTY BACK TOGETHER AGAIN

I'd been lying in a hospital bed for somewhere around three or four months. Every day was a constant parade of people coming in with sympathetic looks. They'd see me laying there and say things full of doom and gloom. "We're *so sorry* this happened to you." "It's such a shame! You had so much promise." "Oh, this is TERRIBLE for you!" Every person: depressed. Every conversation: depressing.

Sometimes they focused on my prognosis: "What did the doctor say?" (Nothing good.)

Sometimes they stated the obvious: "Oh, you can't move! How awful." (No shit.)

Sometimes they poured salt on the wound: "You lost your job?! Oh gosh, and you have so many medical bills to worry about … " (Thanks for bringing it up, jerk.)

It was so much crap to listen to.

One night, around 2:00 a.m., a nurse came in to change my IV. She was gentle and caring as she proceeded to look for a vein that hadn't already been blown. My wrists and hands had been useless for months. I'd had IVs in my feet and in my neck. By the glow of the monitors, she quietly looked all over my body for a new vein. The machines were thrumming and whirring as she quietly asked me one of my least favorite questions: "How are you?"

How was I? A silent rant went through my head: "Well, I might be in a wheelchair for the rest of my life. I might get access to the best possible medication, and the best possible medical care, and it still might not work. There seems to be little to be hopeful about. For months, I have been lying in a bed or sitting in a wheelchair, and I am angry and sad. I feel so mad that I'm never going to walk again. I'm mad at the world. I'm mad at everybody. I feel like nobody wants to be around me. *I* don't want to be around me."

That triggered a new thought. I imagined being home with Stephanie, rolling around our kitchen in my chair. I thought, *What IF I never walk again? What IF I'm in a wheelchair for the rest of my life?* I pictured myself with this same depressing attitude, not talking to her, feeling down and miserable and sorry for myself.

To hell with THAT, I thought.

I changed the picture. I imagined myself in the wheelchair putting food together for us, asking her about her day, looking at her homework with her. I wanted that self to be upbeat, even if I couldn't stand.

I thought, *There's too much life still to live to spend it feeling like this every day. If I have to live this life sitting instead of walking, I won't like it, but I have to choose to make the best of it. I*

*need to make choices that will drive me toward joy and hope. If I
don't, life isn't going to be worth living at all.*

I said out loud, like an announcement, "Well, I'm *done* with
this part."

The nurse startled. "I'm almost done … " she said apologetically, refocusing on the IV.

I stared forward. "Tomorrow, when it's a new day, we are going
to have a new attitude." She murmured some sort of placating
agreement.

I was sick of being sick. I was tired of the expressions of sympathy. Those were fine, up to a point, but they were starting to
hinder my ability to practice acceptance, growth, and evolution. I
was ready to move forward.

The next morning, I told people that they couldn't come see me
unless they followed a strict set of rules. "I'm done with this pity
party," I announced. I told everybody what the rules were going to be:

> "You are only allowed to talk to me about positive things
> that I would normally want to talk about; for example,
> 'How is Stephanie doing in school?'
>
> "You are NOT allowed to ask questions about
> depressing, disease-related things, such as, 'What is your
> long-term prognosis?' (Barf.)
>
> "If you are going to ask me about my disease, ask me
> what *accomplishment* I've experienced today, like,
> 'What is something positive you've done recently?'"

I started embracing humor, especially with people who asked
me dumb questions, like, "How do you feel today?" I would

respond, "I feel great! I can't wait to go run a marathon!" They were feeding me nonsense, so I embraced the absurdity.

Instead of lying in my hospital bed and letting the physical therapist come find me for my mandatory sessions, I asked the aides to push me to the in-house PT clinic. I started *making an effort.* It was brutal—I couldn't do a thing. But six months later, I could. I became religious about going three times a week: I wouldn't let myself cancel and I followed through with the exercises.

It was the same with occupational therapy. For the longest time, I didn't even try. I was insulted by the little grips they gave me to get dishes out of the cupboard from my wheelchair. But acceptance prompted me to do it, try it, use all the tools. The OT therapists also taught me about energy conservation, which was a game changer for me.

My attitude was: I'm done with this. I'm not staying here anymore. I'm going to get out. I told myself, "I'm going to be a mom. I am going to make toast again. I'm going to make a fucking piece of toast for Stephanie, and if I have to do it sitting in a wheelchair, using a gripper tool to get the bread down out of the cabinet and put it in the toaster, then so be it. I'm going to start doing things that normal, non-sick people do."

When I changed my thinking to acceptance, I went from being a reluctant patient to an empowered patient. The shift gave me a higher level of engagement with my healthcare plan. In addition to increasing my PT and OT, I was actively looking forward to the first FDA approval of a new medication for MS that my doctor had told me about. Apparently, the supply of the medication was going to be far lower than the need, but my doctor had entered me into a lottery in the hopes I might be one of the first to receive it. That was something to hope for. I tried a support group. All of that started to make a difference. I was getting stronger. People were responding to me differently.

I got out of the hospital. I moved in with some family members. I *left the house*—which felt like a huge deal. Leaving the house in a wheelchair is like leaving the house with an infant, only *you're* the infant, and you need to recruit somebody else to pack up all the shit and help you get out the door and drive you somewhere. But I was doing it. I decided I wasn't going to be afraid of people seeing me in a wheelchair. I said to myself—and anyone else who would listen—"I need to embrace my life."

It was in the Acceptance stage that I started putting Humpty Dumpty back together again.

CHOOSE YOUR FIGHT

For many patients, the word "acceptance" seems like it implies surrender, somehow. We use war metaphors to describe disease: "I'm battling cancer." "I'm fighting depression."

I knew that I was always going to have to "fight" my MS because one part of my body was literally attacking another part of my body. And that's true for most people living with any kind of chronic or terminal illness: the struggle is real. You must show up to that fight every day—not by choice, but because you *have* to, which can easily cause you to feel like you've lost control over every area of your life. That's one of the reasons why Grief and Anger sweep in so powerfully at first: you feel as if you have no choice over what's happening to your life.

But here's the thing: you don't have to fight *everything*. I had to fight my MS in the hope of getting better, but I was also fighting the fact that I *had* MS, which was leading me into anger, denial, avoidance, and bitterness. That was diffusing my very limited energy and keeping me stuck in negativity. In the Acceptance phase, I recognized that I could choose to stop fighting things I couldn't control. If I chose to accept my diagnosis of MS and make peace with it, I would be better positioned to focus all my fighting energy toward the *one* thing I should be fighting: my disease. That's where my efforts needed to go.

People still in the Anger phase don't want to accept their illness. Accepting it, to them, means letting it win.

I'm suggesting the opposite. I'm saying that by accepting it, *you* win.

You have control over something. You can decide to let go of your sense of victimization, feeling sorry for yourself, and anger. You can accept that this *is* happening to your body and make peace with that fact. When you do that, you conserve your energy and can deploy it for the fight that means the most. You are able to become an empowered patient instead of a passive one when you accept that this disease will be part of your life moving forward.

By accepting that this disease will be part of your life moving forward, you are able to become an empowered patient, instead of a passive one.

I did not make the decision to accept my MS lucidly or strategically. I made it because I finally got too exhausted to do anything else. In the middle of the night, feeling overwhelmed from test after test, dealing with yet another IV needle and blown vein, I simply had to give way. I realized the only way I would be able to function—ever, in my whole life—was by accepting this. I was too tired to keep fighting it.

And when that realization came to me, it was like a switch flipped. In retrospect, I can see that acceptance was my first direct step toward wholeness.

It didn't happen immediately. It's not like the next day I was Suzy Sunshine. But it was after making this mental switch that I found myself with a new mental image of my MS. I pictured it as a little creature—an ugly, pathetic thing. This was my small, sick Me. I couldn't cut her out of my family, because she was me; somehow, we had to work in partnership with each other. The strong, big Me needed to bring her in from the cold. I needed to reach down, hold her hand, and help her cross the street.

Before I accepted my disease, I had viewed MS as something external—a devil, an adversary, an enemy, the weed in the garden. I wanted to kill it or remove it somehow. But that put me at unbelievable odds with myself.

My disease was *part* of me. There was no cure. There was no getting rid of it. I had to accept it so that I could love myself again.

My disease was *part* of me. I had to accept it so that I could love myself again.

I internalized the truth that this little, ugly part of me wasn't going away. And by accepting her, there was an emotional and psychological shift that started to calm everything down in my body—like a big sigh of relief. I took myself out of "fight or flight" mode, with all its waves of cortisol, and tried to help my body calm and heal.

The Patient's Journey is a wild roller coaster ride. As I've shared earlier in this book, the stages will not always be linear, and they'll often loop back on one another. But Acceptance is a stage that *is* more definite. Acceptance enables you to cross a threshold that changes the rest of your Patient's Journey. Every experience that follows Acceptance—even the return of Grief and Anger—is tinged with a new hue of relief. *This has happened to me. This is here. This is mine to deal with.*

Getting through this journey isn't a purely physical odyssey. It's not just about taking the medicine, doing the physical therapy, and so on. It's also a journey of the heart and the mind. *These* things also need to heal.

If you are at war with yourself, how can you heal? By choosing to look at the small, sick part of you and recognize *this is you*, something changes. You are able to move forward when you choose to love this part of yourself. You allow your mind, heart, and body to begin the deep work of healing.

THE CHALLENGE OF ACCEPTANCE

That doesn't make Acceptance easy. MS wrecked my heart and wrecked my soul, in addition to destroying my body.

Prior to Acceptance, our focus tends to be drawn toward everything that has been taken away by this disease. We all envision our lives going a certain way, and disease is the ultimate monkey wrench. It's the ultimate disrupter of all our carefully laid plans! It forces a detour that nothing in your previous life could have prepared you for. When it hits, you are at your most vulnerable, while also feeling completely unprepared. That's a scary place to be.

I'm not suggesting that, in accepting your disease, you love it. It's completely appropriate to say, "I don't like having this disease," but that's different from saying, "I refuse to accept this."

I don't fucking like having MS. However, I *accept* that this has happened to me, and that MS is now a part of who I am. And by internalizing it and accepting it, I'm able to have other parts of me flourish. The best parts of Brenda Snow can grow. I can have hope and choice and wholeness and happiness; I can develop great strategies to manage my MS.

If you can't allow yourself to move forward into Acceptance and make peace with your sickness, the only part of you that will get air and attention is the disease. And then, you are *only* your disease. You're not able to feel hope, which means you're not able to make proactive choices. You're not able to realize that there is another *good* life you can live with illness. Without Acceptance, you're going to continue to churn through anger, fear, and denial, like a hamster on a wheel.

If you can't allow yourself to move forward into Acceptance and make peace with your sickness, the only part of you that will get air and attention is the disease.

So, here's what we're going to do. We're going to take an honest look at all the sucky parts of disease, all the burdens. We're not going to try to paper over them or pretend they don't exist. We're going to say, "Yes. These are here. The disease has caused ugly things to happen in my life and I don't like them."

Then, we're going to balance the scales. After taking an objective look at the burdens, I'm going to walk you through the gifts. I want these gifts to open your eyes to the possibilities before you. We're going to set their weight against the burdens and watch the "gift" side of the scale pull the greater gravity.

The goal is not for you to feel amazing or elated by the end of this chapter, but to simply arrive at a place where you can say, "Okay. This is part of my life now. So, how can I make the best of my time?"

THE BURDENS

Burdens first. (These are not hard to brainstorm.)

Upended Life

Let's start with the obvious: your life has been upended. If you were working, you've probably had to take time off from your job. Your job performance may have been impeded, or perhaps you've even lost your job. For many patients, disease quickly results in financial stress, especially if job loss has jeopardized your health insurance. That's incredibly stressful. These are real barriers to the Patient's Journey; compromised insurance can impede your ability to get the help, medication, and therapies you need.

Losing a career can also cause you to experience a crisis in your identity. You go from being someone who identifies as a contributor to someone who needs to call on family and friends for help. In addition to losing financial stability, you lose your sense of self.

Also, many diseases occur when you're in your most productive years. You might have been family planning or looking for a long-term romantic partner. Maybe you wanted to advance in your career. Although many people *will* go on to experience these things in spite of their diseases, it can be easy to assume that you will lose all the opportunities you had hoped for in life. And that can feel devastating.

Symptoms

Every serious health condition comes with some level of pain or other forms of miserable physical discomfort, whether they're brought on by the disease itself or by medication side effects. That's a real burden. No one can underestimate how much these symptoms impede the body's ability to heal and a person's ability to feel hope and positivity.

Early on, no one talked to me about my pain or discussed ways to manage it. The pain was like a "phantom" thing—it couldn't be real. But there *was* physical pain in my body. There was also emotional trauma.

Eventually, I learned that I had to proactively bring this up in my doctors' appointments and ask them for help managing my physical and emotional symptoms. There are many strategies to help with symptom management—both with pharmaceuticals and non-pharmaceutical interventions—but when your discomfort is chronic, it might not occur to you to even ask. The physical discomfort can start to feel like it's simply a permanent and nonnegotiable part of your life. It won't go anywhere. But until your symptoms are managed, moving forward will be difficult. Another weight on the scale.

Your Body Changes

Sickness changes your appearance. Some patients I know with psoriasis deal with changes to their skin. I gained a tremendous amount of weight from steroids and lost a lot of my muscle tone because I had to be inactive for so long. There are visible symptoms, like the ones that come with psoriasis, rheumatoid arthritis, cancer, and so on, but there are all kinds of invisible changes, too. I remember being unable to read the directions to a board game and couldn't understand them even when someone read them aloud. I was often unable to find the word I wanted to say. These changes caused me to feel ashamed and stupid. I imagined what people must be thinking about me: "Poor Brenda. Not only can she not walk anymore, but disease has made her dumb, too. She can't read a book or track how to play a board game." Many of these changes are not permanent, but when you're in an acute stage of illness, these physical and cognitive changes are commonplace.

And that's heavy. When you don't feel at home in your body, and then can't *recognize* yourself in your body, there's an additional loss to your sense of self. "Who is this? I don't even know who this is."

People Can Be Obnoxious

As a person living with an illness, you may be unfortunate enough to run into some of those people on the worse end of the spectrum of humanity: people who are miserable and downright mean, who say cruel things to you. Some people are genuinely that rude. But more often, people are just clumsily ignorant. I encountered many people who—I knew—truly cared about me but didn't know what to do with my illness. Sometimes they would avoid eye contact. They might pretend they didn't even notice the fact that I was in a

wheelchair. They were just *awkward*. And their awkwardness
conspired with my insecurity, making me perceive that they were
looking down on me—even though they were actually doing their
best not to be rude.

Either from intentional rudeness or unintentional ignorance, this
perception of being looked down upon is another huge burden. It
doesn't matter if it's "real" or not. It *feels* real. It feels as though people
don't care or are deliberately ignoring you. That impression can easily
cause your mind to fill in the blanks with a damaging narrative.

When I was in my wheelchair and Stephanie was younger, kids
on the playground pointed at me. It felt like they were making fun
of me and of Steph. That was devastating to both of us.

Later, when I had made some gains and was trying to reinvent
myself, I sought a way to use a storytelling model in the life sciences
industry. I had seen the power of sharing my story by then. I went
to one of the world's biggest biotech companies and managed to
get a seat at the table with some marketing directors to share some
of my ideas. Very quickly, I was patronized to the point where they
may as well have just patted me on the head. I'll paraphrase their
response: "You're so cute having an idea about a story for sick
people. We know your MS story means a lot to you, but we don't
think there's an opportunity here." It's not like they saw a business
plan or road map; they just assumed I was "the crippled girl." How
could I have the energy or the business sense or intel to start a business? They didn't take me seriously, largely because of my illness.

Physicians thought I must be a hysterical woman, making all
this up. Some of my friends made assumptions that I must be too
tired, too crippled, too infirm to spend time with them, so they
stopped inviting me to get togethers.

I'd like to think there's been a big push to increase awareness and understanding around people with disabilities—and that Snow Companies might have played a part in getting more information about illness and disease into the wider consciousness. But people are going to be people, and sometimes, they will just make you feel lousy. So, set that weight on the scale.

Isolation

A heavier weight on the scale: illness can be isolating and lonely. A huge hope of mine in writing this book is to help you feel *less* alone, and to offer you a friend on this journey. You don't have to stay in a place of isolation.

But for many patients, that's one of the initial burdens. I've spoken with many epilepsy patients and all of them felt enormous isolation early on. The seizures that come with epilepsy often come without warning. Seizures can be devastating and embarrassing, so lots of these folks just sat home alone.

I don't want that for anyone—illness or no illness.

Prevented from Doing the Things You Love

Another burden: it's harder to do the things you enjoy most. For example, with MS, my body is unable, at times, to properly regulate heat. If it's a hundred degrees outside and 90 percent humidity, I'm not going to go to the outdoor picnic, no matter how much I might want to. As you go further down your Patient's Journey, you'll become really in tune with where your breaking points are. That self-awareness is helpful, but it's still a drag to recognize that you simply can't do the sorts of things you used to love doing—and that can contribute to a sense of isolation.

You may not be able to be active the way you used to be. You may not be able to function as a parent the way you'd like. Vacations, hobbies, outings with friends, physical intimacy with your partner, success in your career—all of that may have taken a huge hit.

I don't want to minimize a single one of these burdens. Every one of them sucks.

But acceptance can help. Once you accept your illness, you get better at creative problem solving and advocating for yourself. Shortly after I moved back home from the inpatient ward, I saw my neighbors getting together for some event I hadn't been invited to. I watched them all file into my neighbor's house and felt so incredibly sad.

But these days—after living with MS for over thirty years—I'd open the window and yell out, "Hey! You must have forgotten to invite me! Hang on, I'll be right over!"

I've gotten to that place because of how I've been able to move forward, through the process of acceptance. I've learned: I *am* worth it. I'm entitled to a happy life. I'm not going to let illness or the fear of what others think of me stand in my way. And you shouldn't either. Who the hell cares what they think of you, really?

Acceptance allows you to start a life as the new you. Many of the things you love will return to you in new forms. And, if you can vocally educate some of the people in your orbit about what you can and can't do, they'll learn.

Besides, the people who may pity, patronize, or judge you don't realize what they're missing. They don't know anything about the gifts you're discovering on this journey.

PATIENT PERSPECTIVE: NANCY K., BREAST CANCER

The Serenity Prayer advises me to ". . . accept the things I cannot change, [have] courage to change those things I can, and [seek] wisdom to know the difference." From my biopsy onward, I focused my energies on what I could control by learning all I could about my disease and treatments, and by limiting or *eliminating* stressors in my life (including my crazy executive position). I settled in for surgery, chemo, and radiation with curiosity and patience. I put trust in my amazing medical team and chose to respect my body's limitations. Of course, I was often afraid, and I grieved my losses, but I did not allow these emotions to consume me.

I became very active in my cancer support group and that led me to many positive people and situations. I was featured on our local TV station when Herceptin was approved for early-stage HER-2 breast cancer; invited to model designer jeans at LA Fashion Week (a portion of sales went to HER-2 research); and I spoke at various women's groups. These provided a fun and satisfying bridge from my high-octane career to my new purpose—helping others navigate the cancer journey.

As I rack up the years cancer-free, I am reminded of what my oncologist told me. She said, "This will be the hardest year of your life, and then you will go on to live your life. And you will find many gifts along the way." My life today is full and my gratitude for the gifts has not waned. I would never wish cancer on anyone, but I'm glad it happened to me. My relationships are richer, my focus on health is far greater, and I continue to help others navigate through cancer and terminal diseases.

THE GIFTS

The burdens are there—they exist. There's plenty about disease that is lame and unlikeable. Those weights are on one side of the scale. We're not going to pretend like they're not. But we're also going to look at the gifts on the other side.

Special Glasses

You get a rare, special pair of glasses when you're living with disease. They change how you see the world and make it somehow brighter—more dazzling. You begin to see life as the precious thing it has always been, which you didn't have eyes to see before.

You get a rare, special pair of glasses when you're living with disease. You begin to see life as the precious thing it has always been, which you didn't have eyes to see before.

I had two serious episodes early in my MS journey where I came very close to losing my life. And for me, those experiences focused the lens on how finite our time on earth is. My remaining time to live my best life was *limited*. That gave me new clarity about what priorities I wanted to devote my energy toward.

I wanted more special moments with my daughter. I wanted more memories with my parents. I wanted more belly laughs with my loved ones. Everyone *knows* this is the stuff that really matters—but disease heightens your awareness of it. You somehow gain the ability to be more present in each moment.

In this 24/7 world, there are a million ways to be distracted. One of the best gifts that came with my chronic illness is the realization that I could choose not to be interrupted. It's like we're shown how to exit the Ferris wheel. We're able to pause—be present—recognize the fleeting nature of these special, special moments and choose *not to miss them*.

I know I could have an MS attack at any point that could derail my life. So, I don't wait to go over to my daughter's house and sit on the floor with my granddaughter. I'm living my best life when she and I are putting Legos together for two hours. That's probably one of the most important things I could ever do.

Special glasses: your first weight to counterbalance the burdens on the scale.

Empathy and Patience

Prior to my diagnosis, I did not have empathy in abundance. I may not have even had it in scarcity.

It's different now. I've developed tremendous empathy as a result of going through my Patient's Journey, and I truly believe that tapping into this empathy is one of the main reasons I've been able to achieve the level of success I have. I have cried and felt deeply the stories of hundreds of thousands of patients. Using my own story, I've been able to serve as a vessel to others and help them get to a place of inspiration with their own stories.

Empathy has been an incredibly special gift that MS gave me, and I've heard too many stories over the years to think that my experience is unique. This is a gift that disease amplifies, sharpens, and hones—it can become one of your new superpowers when you accept your chronic disease.

Empathy is a gift that disease amplifies, sharpens, and hones.

Patients also say that they discover a newfound level of patience, both with themselves and with others. All the noise and distractions and hurry that non-sick people get hyper-focused on quiets down. In its place, there's a deeper current of patience.

Patience and empathy—these are rich gifts that expand your ability to love others and enjoy life.

Reinvention

We acknowledged the loss from a life upended—but that's counterbalanced by the gift of reinvention. MS presented me with a plethora of new and different opportunities, which was something I never expected after I was first diagnosed. I'll talk about this briefly here, but I'm devoting an entire chapter to this concept later.

Accepting your illness opens the door to innovation for your life. You're able to say, "Okay … There's probably a different life plan for me with this disease. It's not one I was thinking about a year ago. It's not one I might have thought I wanted. But just because I'm sick doesn't mean that I stop thinking about what kind of person I can become."

Just because you're sick doesn't mean that you should stop thinking about what kind of person you can become.

Ask yourself: What can I do with this disease? Take your eyes off the loss, the liability, the financial stress for a moment. That's still real; your limitations are still real, too. You can mourn that bucket—but set it aside for a minute. There's a new bucket for you to fill. As you accept your illness and come to terms with it, consider how you might *reinvent* what goes into this new life. Yes, there's pain from being severed from your old life, but there's also freedom. You get to decide what the next phase is going to look like. Remember how much power there is in taking back your personal narrative. Own your sick story. You can move yourself toward wholeness when you think about a plan for this new season of your life.

Resilience and Empowerment

If you find yourself clawing your way back to physical strength after it's all been taken away, you feel like a total badass. You develop a huge new appreciation for your resilience and your ability to make positive changes in your life. This is another weight on the "gifts" side of the scale.

Acceptance is a slow process, but it's integral for building resilience. After I had my midnight-IV epiphany, I began moving into acceptance over the next six months. But there was a particular moment when I realized I wasn't feeling as angry as I used to feel and thought, *I might be letting this go.* That moment came when I started taking the MS medication that the FDA finally approved.

I wouldn't have experienced that moment if I hadn't made the choice to reach down and hold the hand of my MS, because *choosing* to take the medication was itself an act of acceptance. If I hadn't gotten to the place of accepting my disease, I would have remained in denial. Instead, I recognized that I *did* need help. My small, sick self needed it. Recognizing that fact led me to pursue and take the FDA approved medication.

And that choice began a positive chain reaction that enabled me to gradually build more resilience and a sense of empowerment.

It was one positive thing I did, and that begat another one. Not only did the medication prove efficacious for me, but it also gave me a greater sense of control. I wasn't so afraid of being blindsided by an MS attack. Taking the therapy made me feel like I was owning my treatment; I was gaining more control over flare-ups. These small decisions collectively helped me start putting myself back together.

That led to greater positivity, which led to greater energy, which led to greater effort in therapy sessions. That led to increased strength, which led to increased progress. All of that led to better choices: it was a positive chain reaction, an upward spiral. That was profoundly empowering and made me realize just how strong I could be.

You Stop Sweating the Small Stuff

A chronic or terminal illness is the ultimate accelerator of your perspective. The trivial stuff doesn't matter anymore. You don't give a rip about things you used to be so concerned about, because you realize that, in the broad scheme of things, these are not worth spending your time or energy on!

The only time I've heard anyone talk about this perspective shift who *wasn't* a patient with a chronic illness was a woman in her seventies. She told me, "I used to put so much energy into stupid stuff. I don't anymore. I wish somebody had told me sooner that I could let it go."

She was in her eighth decade of life—but patients realize this so much sooner!

Prior to MS, I would not let anyone come into my house if it didn't look perfect. No way. Look at me now: when my husband's family came from Australia for a visit, we were going through a renovation. We had no dishwasher, no laundry, no kitchen, and there was random construction junk everywhere. And I was like, "Enjoy your stay!"

What a gift to be so much *less* bothered! To be so much less stressed! To be so much less preoccupied with what other people think! It's a strange gift that disease enables: life gets easier to enjoy and laugh about.

Impact

As you go through this metamorphosis and synthesize these gifts into your life, you also step into the gift of impact. This gift is so significant and profound that it's the focus of the last stage in the Patient's Journey, and therefore gets a chapter of its own. But I want to provide a glimpse of what's to come so that you can balance this tremendous gift on the scale with the burdens.

The gift of impact is twofold: one side of it manifests internally, and the other externally. *Internally*, your journey with disease causes you to plug new coordinates into your GPS for your purpose and your ideas of success. The perspective you've gained from navigating a life with illness means you're able to redesign your current reality and future purpose. "Success" may become less about career highlights and more about experiencing satisfying days with your favorite people. It may mean you recognize a need in the world that you would have overlooked otherwise, and you orient your purpose toward meeting that need.

In my own story, this internal impact meant I gave up building my early career and focused instead on getting well enough to care for my daughter. When I felt well enough, I directed my energy toward encouraging other MS patients by sharing my story, which ended up leading to a completely different career. (More on that, soon.)

You can't help but change as you move through this Journey, and that means you're able to direct your energy and choose pursuits you wouldn't otherwise have chosen had you not been diagnosed with a chronic illness. That's the *internal* form of impact.

But there's an external component, too. Your internal transformation will impact how you treat other people. These new skills and "superpowers" you've gained from being a person living with an illness are ones you can share with other people. As a result, you become someone who sprinkles the world with more empathy, sympathy, love, support, and a greater willingness to help all kinds of people. For me, that was a direct result of having my "special glasses" on and internalizing all of the gifts from my journey.

If I were to summarize all these gifts, it would come down to this: life gets sweeter. When you become suddenly aware that your life has an expiry date on it, you don't want to waste time on the "shoulda, coulda, wouldas." And that's why acceptance is so important. If your time draws near, you don't want a bunch of regret around your inability or unwillingness to accept the presence of disease in your life. You don't want to spend these precious days fuming in anger—looking at the pile of shit. There's *always* a pile of shit, with or without a disease. You don't want to be looking for that.

Open your eyes to the rainbow. Acceptance allows you to notice the sunshine permeating the rain.

Acceptance allows you to notice the sunshine permeating the rain.

HOW TO MOVE INTO ACCEPTANCE

What are some practical ways to usher yourself into this stage? Both patients and care partners can help themselves with these strategies.

- **Reality check:** When you're sick and alone, it's easy to let your mind spin and start forgetting what's real and what's not real. A lot of times, we fill our heads with, "This [terrible thing] is going to happen to me!" But that may not even be part of your disease. Don't let your sickness take on even more power than it already has. Often, our fears are never realized. Remember what's real. Get other people to help you if you need it. Acceptance means facing reality, not the monsters in the closet.

Acceptance means facing reality, not the monsters in the closet.

- **Ask for help when you need help:** Even with finances. In partnerships where the patient's income was a needed component of the household's finances, being unable to work is a major burden. The stress it can cause is unreal. If you need help, do the hard thing of alerting your wider community to your needs. Allow them to show up with soup and fundraising contributions. Accepting your disease becomes easier when you remember you're not alone.

- **Say thank you:** Patients need to remember those two simple words, especially for their care partners. There are research studies that show marriages can fail when partners don't say thank you enough; that's just as true for any close relationship enduring a time of huge stress. Remember: your care partner is on their own journey. They're struggling to accept this massive change in their life as well. Fill up your care partner's cup. Saying "thank you" goes a long way.

- **Talk about acceptance:** Have brave conversations with your people. Ask them, "Are *you* accepting this? How are you handling it?" There's strength in numbers. When you can initiate these conversations with the people you love and trust the most, everyone has to process more deeply. They may respond with a laugh— "I'm not!" And then you'll find yourself digging deeper into your own psyche, driving toward your answer to help them. The process can lead to greater insight and understanding for all of you.

- **Embrace ironic humor:** Don't underestimate the power of grim humor to pull you out of anger and into something vaguely more cheerful. I used to joke with my dad all the time about the shit this disease had taken away from me, and then we would make funny lists of things the disease had *given* to me. (You may have noticed, that's *exactly* what I did with this chapter as well.) When we got to the gifts, I didn't bother trying to be sincere. I'd be like, "Adult diapers! This disease has given me adult diapers. Hell, yes!" Handicapped parking sticker—that was a legitimately good one. I told my dad, "Now I can piss off all the old people when I cut them off in the Target parking lot!" It started as a joke, but it initiated a mindset shift, too. I began to consider that some of these things weren't necessarily bad perks. That drove me to consider more intentionally, "Well—what *are* some of the gifts I've gotten out of this?" All of that helped drive me to accept it.

- **Blue sky:** I'm using this as a verb. In 2024 culture, people call it "manifesting." Or "putting something out into the universe." I call it Blue Sky: it's the concept that the sky's the limit and you're not going to put any limitations on an idea. In my dark humor list-making with my dad, we kept another list of all my impossible Blue Sky goals, which always started out as a joke. *"Become a movie star. Be a book author. Start a company. Win 'Kindergarten Mother of the Fucking Year.'"* It all went on the list. But then I got more serious. "Helping others" went to the top of the list. I had seen enough of the MS community to know most patients were largely without support services and lived in constant doom and gloom. My Blue Sky list items oriented around how I could use my voice to help other people. It stopped being a joke; the list gave me a purpose and vision for a reinvented life.

- **Share your story:** Look for opportunities to share your experiences. This will help you take control of your own narrative and intentionally think through some of the milestones you've already navigated. When I began sharing my story with other MS patients, I realized it was a tangible, actionable thing I could do to help other people—but in retrospect, I can see how powerful this choice was in helping *me* heal. By connecting with other people and repeating my story, it provided value to them, but it held even more value for me. It cemented my acceptance of MS and pushed my healing process forward. Since my diagnosis, I've now shared my story thousands of times. For the first few years, whenever I got to the point in my story where I was so sick in the hospital and Stephanie asked if I was going to die, I cried almost uncontrollably. After a few more years of sharing my story, I still cried at that part but maintained more control. I'll never forget the first time I delivered my story and didn't cry at that part. Upon reflection, I thought, *Well. I guess I'm finally healed.*

Sharing your story helps you take control of your own narrative and intentionally think through some of the milestones you've navigated.

I went on to build a company where patients are given a platform to share their own stories in service of other patients. A huge reason I did that was because of the power I experienced—both to help others and to heal myself—through storytelling. Although all of these strategies can help you move toward acceptance, telling your story might be the most powerful way to move your journey forward.

MESSAGE TO CARE PARTNERS: YOUR ACCEPTANCE

Listen, you need to acknowledge that this disease is happening to you, too. It's hitting you in a different way than your loved one, but it's happening. It's okay to feel sad, to mourn, to feel angry, and to go through all those same emotions. It's normal to feel bad for your loved one, and to also feel bad for yourself.

I won't lie: it's easy to stay in the Grief and Anger phases as a care partner. You play that victim narrative: "This has taken everything away from me. I don't want my life changed or altered. I didn't sign up for this." If you can accept your loved one's illness, you're able to believe a new story: "This is hard, and I'm scared. But I'm going to allow this to change me and trust that we can still find a good life, living with this disease. So, what's the best next step forward?"

Acknowledge your feelings—even the ones you feel ashamed of. You don't have to discuss all of them with your loved one, but you need someone in your life that can hear the good, the bad, and the ugly. You'll fare much better if you can honestly unpack your own pain and fear, and move through that dark valley.

Care partners often feel guilt over these emotions, as though it's selfish to think of how this is impacting their own lives. But it *is* impacting your life, too. That's simply reality. And accepting that reality—with all the messy emotions and upended circumstances that go with it—will ultimately *serve* your relationship with your loved one. It will deliver you both to that other side of Grief and Anger where you're able to sigh, scratch your heads, take hands, and say, "Okay. What's next? Let's figure this out."

TAKE ITS HAND

For me, there was no enlightened moment where I concluded, "I'm going to accept all of this shit." I just got sick and tired of being sick and tired. I was exhausted from putting so much energy into negativity and grief and loss and fear. Both of my parents had drilled an ethos of positivity into me for my entire life, and it was in the Acceptance phase that I finally thought, *I wonder if my parents' advice to "stay positive" will work.*

I finally figured, "Well, I've got nothing else to lose." I had faced the loss of nearly everything that mattered to me—both real and imagined losses. I thought, *Why don't we try something different?*

Choosing to accept my MS was like choosing to reach down and hold its little hand. And once I did, I felt empowered. I had lost control over so much—so many things in my life were now gone. But the one thing I could control was my attitude, my acceptance of this stupid disease.

Acceptance can't simply be a box that you check—"Okay, I accept that I'm sick; tick the box. Can we move on now?" If that's your mindset, you've got more work to do. Acceptance needs to come from a place of authentic truth.

Acceptance also takes time. There will always be days when feelings of self-doubt, fear, anger, or grief grab center stage again and push acceptance to the side. Every time I get another MS attack, familiar feelings of insecurity flood in again. It puts me back at the beginning of the Patient's Journey. But because I've become so familiar with its contours by now, I can travel through it much faster. The timeline is condensed. The first time I navigated the Patient's Journey, I think it took me around three years. Now, it takes me a few days. I build myself back up by remembering the amazing things I've been able to do and the struggles I've already overcome. I cross the threshold of Acceptance for whatever new part of my disease is demanding attention. And every time, I feel that same sigh of relief.

If and when you get to a place of acceptance, everything changes from that point forward. You realize—maybe for the first time since being diagnosed—you are *more* than your disease. You are *more* than the sum of your symptoms. This disease is just a small part of you.

It might take work to get yourself there. Grief and Anger descend like a hailstorm, but acceptance is more like a slow dawn you have to move toward.

The reward of getting there is profound. You get the special glasses and discover a newfound perspective. You see humanity in a brighter, more compassionate, more empathic way. You discover new possibilities for your own reinvention and develop a deeper appreciation for life. Everything starts to shimmer in a way it didn't before. Within this Patient's Journey, you remember that there can still be a good life for you.

Be open to it. Listen for it.

And when you're ready—reach down and take its hand.

STAGE 5 OF THE PATIENT'S JOURNEY: ACCEPTANCE

- *Common emotions: fatigue, resignation, feeling sick of being sick, a desire to experience something more positive.*
- *Common pitfalls: dwelling too long on the burdens, convincing yourself you're somehow "winning" if you stay angry, holding on to a victim mentality.*

- *Your best next step: Face reality (not future fears), embrace dark humor, start employing strategies to construct a "new normal," and seek gratitude. Most of all, remember that accepting your disease means being able to love yourself—even the part of you that's sick.*

PART 2

The Good Life—for the Rest of Your Life

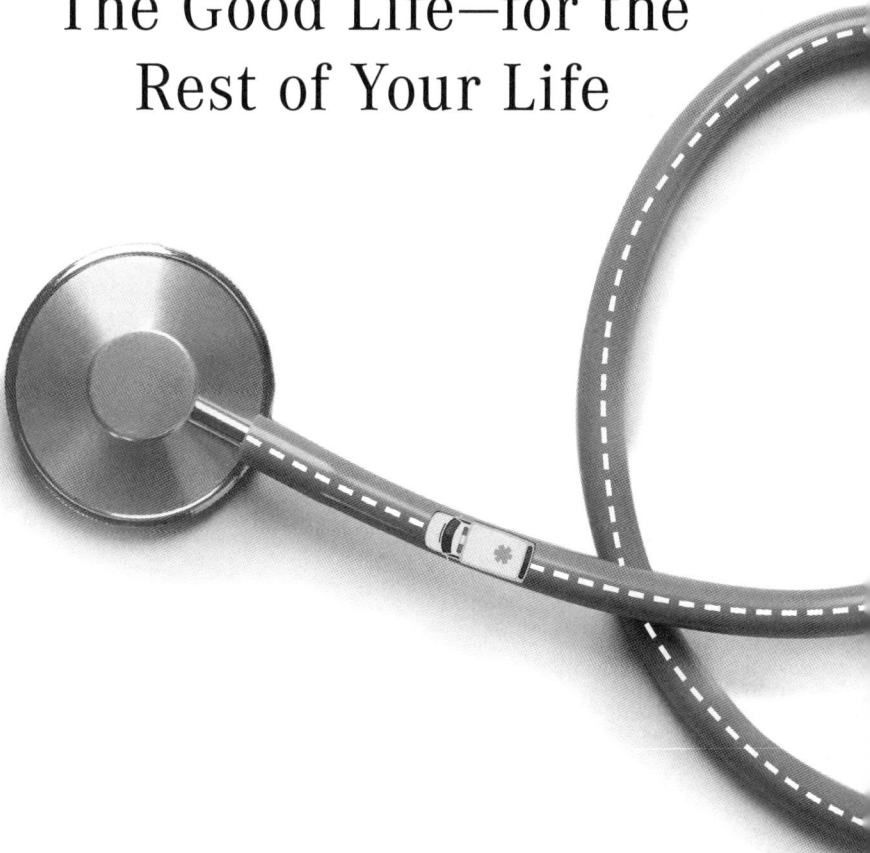

CHAPTER 7

Endurance

HOW TO SET YOURSELF UP FOR THE LONG HAUL

*"To be brave cheerily, to be patient with a glad heart, to stand
the agonies of thirst with laughter and song, to walk beside death
for months and never be sad—that's the spirit that makes courage
worth having."*

— *Sir Ernest Shackleton*

Being able to accept your illness brings you across a crucial
threshold. You've made peace with your diagnosis. You've
begun to redefine who you are and learn your new normal. You're
no longer in constant anger mode and you're not crying every day.
I'd love to tell you that—*ta dah!*—you've finished your Patient's
Journey. But for patients with a chronic or terminal illness, the
"patient" part of the Patient's Journey doesn't go away. Now begins
the long, slow experience of *enduring*.

**For patients with a chronic or terminal illness, the "patient" part of the
Patient's Journey doesn't go away. Now begins the long, slow experience of *enduring*.**

This phase has no end date. You learn to endure your symptoms through each new variation of your illness. You figure out

strategies for endurance, like optimizing your time and available energy. You learn to set clear boundaries and expectations with other people that will allow you to endure well alongside your loved ones. You're solving the questions: How can I do this for the long haul? What changes do I need to implement to ensure I don't burn out, or that my care partner doesn't burn out? How can I make sure I'm devoting my energy to the things that matter most?

It's a retooling phase, a strategizing phase, a strengthening phase. And it's a time when you discover just how resilient you can be.

For me, this phase also coincided with starting on a medication that enabled me to *finally* make some traction against MS's relapses on my body.

TACOS, WITH A SIDE OF BETASERON

In December of 1993, my doctor had submitted my name for the first FDA-approved medication for relapsing MS. Months later, when she finally told me about this, she cautioned me against getting my hopes up. "The manufacturer's original projections were that there wouldn't be enough supply for demand, so they asked us to submit eligible patients' names via lottery," she said. "I didn't think your chances were very high, which is why I haven't told you until now. But it turns out, fewer MS patients want to try this medication than they thought."

I was in disbelief. "Why *not*?!"

"It's new," she said, shrugging. "And for some people, new means uncertain. It's pioneering a new type of treatment called 'biologic therapy,' and it's the first of its kind for MS. Some MS patients have a progressive form of MS, for which the drug has not been approved at this time. But for your condition, relapsing MS, it shows benefits. I think you should try it."

"I'll take it!" I said. "I want it!"

She paused. "Maybe you'll get lucky."

This remark dampened my initial excitement. "I'm the unluckiest person I know," I quipped.

My doctor grimaced apologetically. "Yup."

"So, now I've got to hope to win the lottery to get this medicine?" I repeated. My parents' voices sounded in my brain: *Stay positive.*

On Friday, June 17, 1994, I was watching the news on TV. It was a big night for news: O.J. Simpson was careening down the LA freeways in his white Bronco, leading the LAPD on a wild goose chase. I had moved in with family members after getting out of the hospital because I wasn't able to live independently yet, and Fridays were taco night.

As a California girl taking a lot of steroids and trying to look on the bright side, there was *nothing* I liked more than a good taco. I was happily munching on my tacos, watching that white Ford Bronco on the news in disbelief, and then I was handed a letter. I opened it.

You have been approved to take Betaseron.

I WON THE LOTTERY.

I yelped with glee. "I finally *have* won the lottery!" I called out to the rest of my family. "I get the drug! AND I get tacos! I get the drug and the tacos ON THE SAME DAY!" We all celebrated. I was so excited!

The TV news was showing footage from the helicopters, following the Bronco, and zooming in. I thought to myself, *I have MS and I'm still in a wheelchair, but it could be worse. At least I'm not* that *jackass.*

Everything seemed to be looking up.

It was around that time that I became a manic consumer of everything that even hinted at improved health for my condition. Every library book, every handout, every complementary therapy—if it had *anything* to do with a neurodegenerative disease or multiple sclerosis, I was going to read it and maybe even do it. I was also attending physical therapy three times a week. Along with Betaseron, I lined up everything I could to get myself stronger.

Over the next six months, some of my MS symptoms started to remit—and that was massively, massively uplifting. All the work was paying off. *I was improving.* Before 1994 came to a close, I was hell-bent on graduating from a walker to a cane.

It turns out, getting on that drug as early as I did might have ended up being an enormous blessing. Some of the more current research suggests that if you treat early enough, you can possibly alter the disease's progression. For me, getting treatment early seems to have helped my long-term trajectory. Granted, taking the medication was only one piece of my arsenal to combat MS, and it didn't negate the need to also be diligent about my PT, my OT, and overall looking after my health.

I had accepted that it wasn't my fault that I'd gotten the disease—that's true for *all* patients—but it *was* my responsibility how I dealt with it. (Which is *also* true for all patients.)

You're not responsible for your disease, but you *are* responsible for how you deal with it.

I was developing strategies to endure this illness for the rest of my life.

When the acute symptoms finally abate, patients with a chronic or terminal illness face an indefinite amount of time in which they must learn how to *endure*. This phase is less emotional than many others. It's more strategic. And it lasts a long, long time.

THE ENDURANCE PHASE

By now in your Journey, you've developed a plan to deal with your symptoms. You've gotten medication on board, figured out your ancillary therapies, cultivated a positive mindset, and have begun to figure out your new normal.

But inevitably, there will be setbacks. There will be bumps in the road. Throughout your journey, you might have to revisit therapists or pivot to a new medication or institute. The playbook doesn't necessarily stay the same; you might need to run a new play.

That's why endurance becomes important.

We could swap out several different words for this phase: you must *tolerate* your symptoms. You must *retool*. You need to learn to *advocate* for yourself and others. But I think *endure* is the word that best summarizes the long season that comes in this phase of the Patient's Journey. It's at this stage that you begin to learn how to live your best life with disease. You work at your action plan, hammer at your legacy, and build toward your wholeness.

In the Endurance phase, you work at your action plan, hammer at your legacy, and build toward your wholeness.

Endurance is multifaceted:

- **You need *personal* endurance in terms of dealing with your symptoms.** You will have ups and downs, good days and bad, flare-ups and progress milestones. There will be times when you think, *Oh shit. Is this back? Is it getting worse?* Both physically and emotionally, you must endure this roller coaster ride within your own body.
- **You need *processes* for endurance.** It's important to have systems that help you navigate the healthcare system, your self-care, your boundaries, your division of labor at home, and so on. New and honed routines need to be developed.
- **And you need to endure alongside your *people*.** Learning how to care for your relationships even as you don't feel well is a skill that has to be developed and honed, so that you can endure together with your loved ones.

By devoting attention to all these different areas and learning how to optimize each category, you're crafting your story toward wholeness.

PERSONAL ENDURANCE

Self-care as a term is very "buzzwordy" right now, but it's a non-negotiable for anyone dealing with a chronic or terminal illness.

For example, in the last few months, I've had a few bumps and glitches with MS flare-ups. I've had to go back to some of the self-care practices that I know work: I get extra sleep, I conserve my energy, I call up my doctor, I have conversations with my partner about how to shift our responsibilities. I know how to manage my symptoms and manage my boundaries. Those are the kinds of steps you need to learn to take in order to help yourself endure on a personal level. For patients, self-care could be categorized into three buckets. There's the "symptom management" bucket, where you're working to *mitigate* issues in your body. There's the "proactive physical care" bucket, which is more about *staying ahead* of symptoms by taking care of yourself. The third bucket is *"emotional* self-care," which—if you've heard me talk about hope, positivity, or crafting an optimistic narrative—is vital.

Symptom Management

Let's discuss bucket number one: symptom management. In the early days of your diagnosis, your healthcare team will be most focused on managing your disease. In my case, my doctor gave me steroids to fight the inflammation as when I was diagnosed there were no approved therapies for MS. Later on, I took Betaseron and then Rebif to fight the disease.

But I also had plenty of other symptoms that were ancillary to the disease itself: I had debilitating fatigue and spasticity, I had gotten incredibly weak from all my days in the inpatient rehab ward, and so on. Part of working to get myself better involved speaking up about those symptoms so they could be effectively addressed as well. I needed medications for my bladder, my spasticity, and my fatigue. I also needed to continue PT for strength and occupational therapy to help with my activities of daily living.

Because your symptoms won't typically be the main focus of your healthcare team, they may not think of offering therapeutics to address them. But you need help in this area! How can you expect to make progress with your disease if you feel miserable all the time? Getting help for your symptoms means you will feel more equipped to do all the other hard things on your Patient's Journey.

Therefore, don't suffer in silence. It's up to you to communicate about your symptoms and ask for help. You don't just have to *endure* symptomatic discomfort. The *endurance* required for this category is more about paying attention to your body, having the vulnerability and courage to speak up about your symptoms, and pushing for help.

Endurance in this area also means you need to *keep paying attention* to your body, because your symptoms will change over time. When living with illness, you must get incredibly in tune with your body, especially because it's changed. You don't feel the way you used to feel. "Normal" is not normal anymore, so you have to relearn your body's cues.

Cut yourself some slack as you endure the trial and error of building awareness about when your body feels "normal" and when it feels "off." I did not *really* know my MS body until I'd been living in it for about seven or eight years. For the first five years, I remained in a fairly acute state. I had lots of attacks that followed hard, one after another. But eventually, I began to recognize what was par for the course. I learned that a mixture of good days and bad days was typical; the returning symptoms didn't necessarily mean I was getting worse. It was just my new normal. I also learned to recognize bigger changes in my body that indicated a progression or change in my disease. Those were my cues to sound the alarm and explore new therapies with my healthcare team.

Cut yourself some slack as you endure the trial and error of learning your new body's cues.

Symptom management will eventually become second nature to you. You can speed up the process by paying close attention to how you're doing day to day. I think I may have recommended journaling in every one of these chapters so far, and I'm going to do it again here: keep a log—either electronically or in written format—to monitor your symptoms. You'll start to see patterns that would have otherwise escaped you. A lot of Crohn's patients recognize ways they can avoid certain foods and eat small, frequent meals to lessen their symptoms. You'll start to make helpful connections that teach you about the new body you're living in.

In any case—lining up the right medications and therapies for effective symptom management requires that you *know* what symptoms you have and that you take proactive steps *to address them*. Work with your healthcare team to plan medications, therapy, and strategies to manage your symptoms—not just your disease.

Proactive Physical Care

Which brings me to bucket number two: proactive physical care. This one is fairly straightforward—also known as the "Oh, yeah, DUH" category. You've always known these are ways to take care of your body, but now it's quite urgent that you put them into practice: Eat nutrient-dense food. Avoid foods that cause inflammation or are heavily processed. Get good sleep. *Rest* during the day. Exercise to build strength and maintain energy. Do it with that goal in mind, but don't kill yourself. Be reasonable.

A lot of this stuff is common sense; you hear it all the time, even if you haven't been diagnosed with a disease. But—especially when you *have* a disease—the struggle to actually implement these healthy practices is real. Who doesn't want to binge-watch shows and munch Doritos when you're feeling lousy? Who doesn't want to go out and split a bottle of wine on occasion? But in your case, you will need to be more mindful of maintaining healthy lifestyle practices than the average person to stay ahead of your symptoms. For instance, for my MS, I have to get a *minimum* of eight hours of sleep. I prefer nine. If I don't, everything is much harder.

So, try to work some nutrient-dense recipes into your meal rotation. Put yourself to bed early. When you have the strength to do physical therapy, *do* the physical therapy. Ideally, you want to keep yourself as fit as you can so that you have strength to pull from on the bad days.

Emotional Self-Care

I've already shared a number of strategies to help you fill bucket number three, but it's important to remember that these are practices you need to *continue* doing. The Endurance phase is about *sustaining*. It's about setting yourself up for the long haul. Even after getting out of the most acute phases of your illness, you will still be vulnerable. You will still have days defined by grief and anger. You will still need to fight to claim a positive narrative for yourself. So, *continue* to journal. *Continue* to do things that bring you joy, to the best of your ability. *Continue* to check in with people you love and who make you laugh.

The Endurance phase is about *sustaining* healthy practices that will set you up for the long haul.

And let go of needless pressure. As you get used to living in your new body, it's important to be honest with yourself and recognize you simply can't push your body the same way you did before getting sick. Let go of the guilt you might feel from not doing it all. *Don't* push yourself. Think of this in terms of stewardship: you have a limited amount of energy, and you need to budget that energy for the stuff that counts the most. My occupational therapists taught me about energy conservation early on. The idea is that you save your energy for the things that add value to your life and bring you joy. If you've only got so much energy, use it to build connections in your relationships. Don't expend energy on getting the laundry done. The laundry's going to be there tomorrow! And the next day, too. WHO CARES ABOUT THE LAUNDRY? Let the pressure of these less important things fall away.

Use your good hours for the things that are most important for your mental, emotional, and physical health. Invest in joy. Connect with your people. Do your favorite hobby. Engage in activities that remind you you're *more* than just a sick person. This is how you care for your body and your emotions.

Use your available energy to invest in joy. Connect with your people. Do your favorite hobby. Engage in activities that remind you you're *more* than just a sick person.

PROCESSES FOR ENDURANCE

Your endurance will also be helped along by developing systems or processes in your life that keep things running smoothly. For instance: learning tricks and mindsets to push past roadblocks like healthcare delays or insurance confusion. Or shuffling household responsibilities: if you're not doing the laundry anymore, then who is? Intentional conversations need to be had with those in your orbit to rebalance responsibilities. Set and clarify the new expectations. Figure out the new processes. Sketch out the retooled "standard operating procedures."

If you don't intentionally recraft the processes of daily life, you either cause exhaustion for you or create resentment and frustration for people in your orbit. But by identifying and communicating around these new routines, you can protect your energy *and* your relationships.

Push Past the Roadblocks

After getting through the acute early days of my MS diagnosis, I sometimes woke up feeling good. I'd be like, "Okay, let's go! I'm ready to endure!" No sooner would I put on my big girl pants to do something hard than I'd run into some demoralizing roadblock: "What do you mean I can't get the appointment? What do you mean I'm not covered for an MRI? What do you mean I don't qualify for disability?" It was like getting punched in the face—a game of constant roadblocks. It was *very* hard to endure so many of the tangible, tactical aspects of arranging my medical care or financial coverage.

And this is true for nearly everyone trying to navigate today's healthcare world. In 1993 and '94, I thought healthcare was slow. But it's nothing compared to today. Early on, you're going to be faced with a lot of paperwork, roadblocks, and other crap. In fact, many people *put off* making necessary appointments because the thought of dealing with the inevitable headaches makes it challenging to even begin. In my own Patient's Journey, I was over the Endurance stage long before it ended. But what can you do? What can any of us do other than embrace the suck? The roadblocks will be there whether we like them or not. And that's why this is a point of endurance. Patients today have to have a huge amount of endurance dealing with roadblocks because it takes a long time to get appointments or tests scheduled. The insurance climate is always changing: one minute your drug is approved, and the next month, your pharmacy tells you you're no longer covered. When you're sick and tired, these obstacles are more than an annoyance. They make you want to give up completely. But don't! *Expect to endure.* You can try to make it just a little less sucky for yourself if you use these tips:

- **Enlist professional help.** Find a nonprofit that can help you, or if you can financially afford a lawyer to help you work through forms, insurance appeals, and so on, I recommend it. Professionals can provide invaluable help in navigating some of the complex logistics of your finances and care.
- **Keep your records together.** Know where your test results are. Back in my day, that meant I literally brought a large banker's box of file folders to each appointment with my latest test results. I also demanded to have my own copy of each new document regarding my care. It's slightly easier to keep track of records now that most medical appointments have a digital record, but don't

take it for granted that all your records are digitized on some universally shared database among your doctors. Even with the progress that's been made in digitizing medical records, it's still easy for things to fall through the cracks in the shuffle between hospital systems and specialists. *You* need to get your own system in place for compiling and organizing your medical records. If your doctor wants to send your results directly to the specialist, ask to be cc'd on those emails. You are entitled to have your own records. Keeping them consolidated and handy gives you that safety net in case one of your care providers doesn't pay enough attention.

- **Expect to get denied disability benefits at first.** *Most* people get denied at first, and I was no exception. After getting multiple denials and dealing with no income for close to a year, I finally went to the National MS Society and asked if they had anyone on a legal team who could help me navigate it. They gave me a referral to someone who was able to tell me, "This is what we need to do," and helped me reapply. Finally, I was able to get the benefits. Once I was able to work again and didn't need the benefits anymore, I stopped them.
- **You can often be seen sooner by calling and asking about cancellations.** If you can't get an appointment or a necessary test as soon as you need to, try calling every morning to ask if there have been any cancellations. Calling this often requires endurance too, obviously, but it's a way to be seen much sooner than you would have been otherwise.

All of these steps are hard, and the challenges are magnified when you don't feel well. The sad truth is that there will always be some people who fall through the cracks. The patients who are successful are either totally kickass, enlist professional help, or have a tenacious and proactive care partner. Be encouraged though: endurance *does* get easier as you feel better.

Many of the other processes you need for endurance are relational in nature. One of the most important processes to develop early on is *boundary setting*.

Boundary Setting

Get really comfortable with the word "no." This is a mantra I use a lot: "No" is not a dirty word.

"No" is not a dirty word!

(And I know a thing or two about dirty words!) On my own journey and from talking to many other patients, I've learned that "no" is deeply necessary. Allow me to demonstrate:

"Would you like to come to wine country with us this weekend?"

"That sounds lovely, but no."

"Our meeting time has ended, but there are still a few points to discuss. I can stay late. Can you?"

"No, I need to wrap it up here."

"We're moving and I've enlisted friends and family to help me pack up. Would you mind joining us this weekend? Pizza provided."

"I would love to help out, but I'll have to pass, sorry." (Sometimes, being seriously ill can be a welcome excuse!) Embrace "no"! Get over feeling like you've let people down. There are *so* many things I've had to pass on to stay optimal. If I've worked four long days in the office and didn't sleep a couple of nights, I cannot plan a weekend full of activity. I need to tell my people, "Look, it's not a good time for me. I thought I was going to be able to make it, but my body is telling me I need to just spend a chill day close to home." By recognizing your limits and asserting your ability to say no, you will protect your energy in necessary, important ways.

Boundary management extends beyond your calendar activities. In this Patient's Journey you're living out, people will start to reveal new sides of themselves that escaped your attention before. Some people may reveal themselves to be incredibly unhelpful. Others may simply be irritating. Others may be a drama drain, sucking up energy with negativity or volatile emotions. Sometimes, these challenging people may be in your own family. And when you're in an acute state with your symptoms or jacked up on medications, your tolerance for difficult people is much lower.

So, if there is a person in your life causing you excessive stress, you've got to neutralize the situation. You are allowed to distance yourself from this person. Just as you need to get comfortable with the word "no," you need to get comfortable stating your boundaries. You can graciously "ghost" a negative person, avoid them, or simply be upfront and tell them you need distance—which is probably the best approach.

I want to acknowledge that this is much easier said than done. It's easy to *say* you're going to set boundaries. It's much harder to actually tell your friend you need to take some space from the relationship. Boundary setting is hard because it requires you to be vulnerable at a time when you're already feeling insecure. You don't feel like yourself. You've been sad, angry, depressed, and exhausted. You feel like you've been a bad friend, spouse, parent, [fill in the blank] already and you don't feel fun anymore. So, the last thing you want to do is alienate people who are trying to love you.

At the same time, your energy *is limited*. And if you've got an "energy suck" person in your life, or you have acquaintances coming by for the first time in three years, apparently to bear witness to your sad situation—there's a need for a boundary! This process is not easy, but it's necessary.

So, one of the ways you can make this process slightly easier is by taking a smaller step. If you're not ready to draw hard boundaries, provide *feedback* to continue the relationship in a healthier way.

Provide Feedback

Another variation of boundary setting involves giving clear feedback. This is especially important for people you want to *keep* in your orbit but who need to be reeducated about what's helpful. There will be a lot of well-wishers who come by when you're sleep-deprived or anxious or feeling lousy, and they're going to say some crazy-ass stuff. Your family will do things that annoy the hell out of you. Really, there's no shortage of ways people can cause you to feel insane.

So, as nicely and calmly as you can, give them feedback. I've discovered it's relatively easy to say, "I know you mean well, but that's not helpful. Let me tell you how you can help me." They will get the message. And my advice is to do that early on—the earlier the better. That way, the irritation doesn't build, and they learn what they can do to *actually* be helpful.

It's relatively easy to say, "I know you mean well, but that's not helpful."

There was an encounter I had with my neighbor once where I had to steer the conversation in this direction. At the time, I was living at home and trying to graduate from a walker to a cane. I was also dealing with chronic fatigue. Anyone who has ever experienced chronic fatigue knows that it is no fucking joke. It's nothing close to regular fatigue. But my neighbor didn't know that.

On this particular day, I was trying to walk from my front door to the mailbox. My house was on a teeny, tiny lot—classic for California. You could plug in the lawn mower inside the house and still mow the entire lawn. The distance from the front door to the mailbox was less than ten yards. But for me—with my cane and my chronic fatigue and my shaky legs—it felt like the length of a football field. By the time I reached the mailbox, I was *done*. I was done in a way I still can't even get my head around.

The neighbor lady across the street must have seen me slowly make my way to the curb and she popped outside. She was peppy. She was still wearing her tennis clothes. She volunteered for all the things—in fact, she was probably a regular chaperone for school field trips for her three kids. She smiled and called across to me, "How are you?"

I said, "I'm really fatigued."

She said, "Oh, I *know*. I know, I am so tired, too." Then she proceeded to give me a litany of things that had made her tired: She had been shopping. She had rushed the kids to all their extracurriculars. Her in-laws were visiting, so she was trying to clean the house. I was wobbling on my legs, barely able to stand. I knew she assumed that our fatigue was the same—and her comments were probably made in an effort to connect with me. She was trying to empathize. But she just had no idea.

I jokingly said, "Maybe 'tired' is not the right word for the kind of fatigue I'm experiencing. Because of my MS, it feels like somebody's drilled a hole in the top of my head and filled my body with half-settled concrete. So, I'm a person with half-settled concrete trying to get from my mailbox to the front door."

I could see her expression change. "Woah," she said. "I'm sorry."

I said, "You don't have to be sorry. I just wanted to tell you what that fatigue feels like for me. Because I've also been tired as a mom, before MS. And in no universe do they compare. They're just two very different things."

She nodded. I attempted to smile and wave, then turned around to make the long trek back to the front door. I barely made it, then I fell asleep for three hours. Like I said: I was *done.*

But I had communicated something necessary to my neighbor. And she had a lot more sensitivity after that about what was really going on with me.

You need to advocate for yourself as much as you can on this Patient's Journey. Embrace your inner ballbuster. Get clear about your needs and about what you'd like to happen. Do that as much as you can from day one, and on the acute flare-up days, when any sort of self-advocacy feels impossible, recruit your care partner to be a ballbuster for you.

Advocate for yourself as much as you can on this Patient's Journey.
Embrace your inner ballbuster!

Provide feedback to your healthcare team as well. Your Patient's Journey will go more smoothly when people around you understand clearly how your illness feels and how you're navigating it. If you like your healthcare team and they're doing great, but then you leave an appointment feeling confused or unsettled—provide them with feedback. Call them or email them: "Hey, when you said this, it made me feel confused about X, Y, and Z." Close the feedback loop on what didn't work for you so that it doesn't happen again. And certainly, if your doctor persistently treats you in a dismissive way, get the hell out of there. Find a healthcare team who respects you enough to give you the explanations and care you deserve.

The goal of feedback is not purely to help you personally, although that's a big part of it. You also have a *mission* to do this, to make things better for patients everywhere. If you can share with people what it looks like to be sick and paint the picture of what's happened to you, you help open people's eyes. You broaden their understanding of what's helpful and what they can do for others in a similar situation. And you let other patients know that they're not alone! This is why Snow Companies puts such an emphasis on patient stories. If it didn't work and the stories weren't helpful, I wouldn't have a successful business. Educating others, sharing your stories, being clear about how people can help—these things *work*.

Here's the point: you want to diminish the unnecessary noise. You've got enough on your plate to deal with already. Wherever you can neutralize an area that wants to suck up your precious, finite energy—do it. Make things as easy on yourself as you possibly can.

Diminish the unnecessary noise. Make things as easy on yourself as you possibly can.

Division of Labor

Living long term with illness also means that there needs to be a reshuffle of responsibilities. You may not be able to function the same way you used to at work. At home, it's the same story: maybe you used to do the yard work, cooking, vacuuming, or what have you—but now your capacity is more limited. That's why another key strategy for the Endurance phase is to have discussions with your colleagues and family members about division of labor.

When my MS starts simmering, my vision wobbles. I struggle to read directions or perform visual cognitive tasks—I have to process everything by hearing it. That means my husband has to do nearly all of our administrative stuff, particularly when it comes to filling out forms; reading and systematically following directions can be challenging for me. And as a result, we have to rethink our division of labor around the house. I have to tell Oliver, "I'm going to need your help on this." And bless him, he does a Herculean amount for us.

Have these intentional conversations. I've seen too many patient stories where partners experienced pent up consternation because they never discussed "division of labor" issues. It's not uncommon in families for everyone to have "their lane." One partner does the budgeting and all the big chores inside the house; the other partner handles the kids' activities, makes the appointments, and does all the chores outside. The kids are responsible for homework and their chores. Everyone's got their lane.

But once again, "normalcy" is upended by disease. There may be a whole host of tasks you're not able to do anymore and you've got to enlist the help of the other people in the home to rebalance who does what. This should be a conversation the whole family engages in: everyone needs to say, "Here's what I can do. Here's what needs to be done. Here's who's going to do it, and here's how frequently we're going to do it."

If you're still working at your job, and you realize there are certain tasks you won't be able to do for a time—or may not ever be able to do again—set up a conversation with HR. Ask for a reasonable accommodation; they are legally obliged to work with you and your healthcare provider to make this accommodation. I can think of stories from patients who often struggle with their symptoms early in the morning—that might be the case for someone struggling with rheumatoid arthritis, for instance—so a later start time would be warranted. Another reasonable accommodation might be redistributing responsibilities among your team, so that the tasks assigned to you are ones you can confidently do.

The patient shouldn't do *nothing*. Even us sickies want to add value and contribute! I always encourage families and friends to look for ways the patient can still help out, unless their illness makes that absolutely physically impossible. At home, for example, one of the things I could always do was fold the laundry. On many days, I couldn't physically walk to the laundry machine and back, but I could lay in my bed and fold. I could sit on the sofa and fold.

Get honest with yourself; look at what you still can do. Identify the things you *want* to do and identify where you'll need someone else to pick up the slack.

When you do this, you'll discover two things. First, you'll find you were underutilizing a lot of your household talent! Kids can do more than we usually let them do and other people in your sphere will also rise to the occasion. Second, you'll realize that a lot of the things you were worrying about are not worth your time. *Nobody* needs to do them because it's not a big deal.

How do you know which things you don't have to worry about? Easy: get sick. You will suddenly have amazing clarity about the pointlessness of regularly dusting the baseboards: "Gosh, that was kind of stupid to spin out about. I can get it done whenever I get it done, and that's fine."

Embrace help from your wider network as well. When you're in an acute place with your illness and struggling to manage household functions, lean into your extended community. Accept the meal train offers—if not for yourself, then for your family members. Delegate household tasks to your family and friends. Get a plan in place for who's going to drive the kids to their lessons and pick them up.

These are hard phone calls to make—believe me, these might be some of the *hardest* calls to make. I've heard patients tell me a million times, "I can't ask; I don't want to bother them … " But it's not a bother! Most of the time, there are other parents going to the same place anyway. Who's in your kid's soccer club? Who else is in the ballet class? Just ask.

Here's the beauty of all this: I guarantee you—having experienced this Patient's Journey firsthand—you will have *plenty* of opportunities to pay them back. I've been fortunate enough to help everyone who ever helped me. And it's a joy. People feel gratified when they are able to help someone else! You'll feel good about it when it's your turn, and in the meantime—while it's *you* in the hospital gown—you can give others an opportunity to feel good by helping you. (And let's be honest: you could use it!)

Remember: the most important aspect of the "division of labor" conversations is simply to *have them*. You can't eat an elephant in one bite; you need to be aware of your limits and communicate what those are. Flex your access to resources when needed—let people help you when they offer.

And then, *keep* having the conversation. As you feel better, tell your crew you're able to do more. As you have flare-ups or bad stretches, tell them you're going to have to do less.

The most important aspect of the "division of labor" conversations is simply to *have them*. And then, *keep* having the conversation.

Which brings me to our last category of Endurance: enduring alongside your people.

PEOPLE ENDURANCE: SETTING YOUR LOVED ONES UP FOR THE LONG HAUL

Let's hope your illness has caused you to realize just how much you need other people in your life to help you stay afloat. We will discuss in detail how important relationships are on your Patient's Journey in the next chapter, but right now, one thing I'd like for you to understand is that *their* endurance is *your* endurance.

And this is no small thing. Most care partners find themselves suddenly in that role—whether they're the lover, spouse, best friend, parent, or close relative of someone who becomes gravely ill. Care partners are inclined to practice the same denial that patients do in the Pre-Diagnosis phase: "It won't be for long. I love this person. I made my commitment. I'm in this and I'm sure this part will be over soon."

When the illness turns out to be a much bigger deal, care partners have a choice to make about whether or not they're going to see this through. For some care partners, this isn't a question. Parents, in particular, tend to not even view this as a choice. But other care partners have a tough decision to make. If their sick person *never* gets over it—will they endure in the care partner role? Can they *keep* choosing this life?

MESSAGE TO CARE PARTNERS: YOUR ENDURANCE

I'm going to call out the elephant in the room and be brutally honest: You're not the sick one.

Your loved one doesn't have a choice about living with sickness. You do.

I recommend that you open your eyes wide and comprehend the changes that are happening. Can you stick with this? Can you endure for as long as it lasts? First of all, know that you probably have more endurance than you realize—many, many people grow in profound ways during a care partner experience and muster strength they never realized they were capable of. But other times, care partners hurt the patient by continuing in the relationship with a half-hearted or resentful spirit. When that happens, one of the most important relationships in the patient's life becomes filled with drama and conflict. That helps no one; it makes a hard situation much, much worse.

Instead, make up your mind to *do* this for the long haul and adapt the advice in this chapter for yourself. You must practice self-care. You must engage in figuring out new processes to make this life work. You must communicate and be vulnerable with your loved one. You need to seek out a community that fills up your cup.

Endurance requires work. It's hard to maintain the positive mindset you need unless you practice deliberate self-care. You need to have *your* needs met too. You need breaks and time away to "do you," so that you don't burn out and leave. Endurance means you're running a marathon, not a sprint.

If you don't take care of *yourself* in the role of care partner, you won't be able to take care of your loved one. And then it's just a matter of time before all the wheels come off the cart and you break down. What happens then? Your loved one is worried about *you*.

Remember: as long as you function in this role of care partner, give yourself permission to take breaks. Go down to the pub and have a pint with your friend. Book a massage. Schedule a coffee date. Set up a standing pickleball match. Other people in your household need these breaks, too. Teenage kids of patients need to go out and be with their friends. Young kids need play dates and activities. The patient will be okay lying in bed and resting for a few hours while you're gone.

These sorts of practices will help you endure this illness in a sustainable way. Failure to care for yourself in practical ways can be fatal to the relationship. Only by building a sustainable lifestyle that allows you to endure can you move forward into a satisfying life that includes your loved one's illness.

Finally, work on your communication with your loved one. Without that shared communication and teamwork, you're going to struggle to achieve the good outcomes you want. But vulnerable conversations can generate trust, strength, and love. Work together as a team on all of the concepts discussed in this book.

Care For the People in Your Orbit

Because of the challenge that care partners face, patients need to understand the importance of proactively caring for the people who support them.

Granted, your level of contribution to others will depend on where you're at in your disease and your energy level. But still, it takes little energy to tell someone, "Thank you." Or "I appreciate you so much."

It takes little energy to tell someone, "Thank you."

Another low-energy strategy I've been able to use throughout my ups and downs has been to *remember* what people tell me. You'll have little conversations with people as they bring you a meal or check in with you. Do your best to ask how *they're* doing and then remember what they tell you. When I come across an article I know Susan would love, I take a picture of the article and send it to her. If I come across a great gardening podcast and I know Jim and Becky are starting a garden, I'll text them the link. When I see A.J., I ask if she was able to figure out her dog's limp. These are simple ways you can show people, "You matter to me. I listen to you enough to know that you have an interest in this.

I'm paying attention to what's important to you, because you're important to me."

One tick further up on the energy scale would be to connect with people through handwritten notes. I have little personal stationery that I use to write to people when I'm thinking about them, and I think people enjoy getting a handwritten note in the mail. Particularly if you're experiencing isolation because you're homebound or in treatment, you can use these little work-arounds to stay connected. Facetime or video messages are also helpful when you can't be with someone physically.

And when you *can* rally to do something that requires more physical energy to care for people in your orbit, keep it simple. Gone are the days when I used to host a party and planned to handle all the cooking, cleaning, and decorating by myself. Now, if I want to have a gathering, I do a potluck. Or, I'll delegate a cooking crew and a cleaning crew. There's some beauty in leaning on community and experiencing the ways everyone pitches in. You don't have to overengineer it. Keep it simple.

When it comes to your care partner, help them get out and have fun. It's hard work to be a patient's main support, even if there's nothing they'd rather do. In order for them to continue serving you with love and energy, they need breaks. They need you to tell them that it's *okay* to have a life that isn't solely focused on you. Encourage them to go for a hike or a run or a walk. Don't balk if they mention getting together with a friend. If they're considering therapy, support it. You can even help facilitate these breaks. I encourage Oliver to go out with his friends or take the flying lessons he's been talking about. I know that if he gets out of the house, it will be good for both of us. You can help your care partners schedule these breaks on the calendar. In all these ways, you're helping the both of you endure this Journey for as long as it lasts.

Also, risk vulnerability with your care partner—and, even more importantly, invite it from them. As close as your patient/caregiver relationship might be, I've found that patients and care partners sometimes wonder if the other understands what they're going through. In order to understand each other in a meaningful way, be honest about the fact that you are *both* vulnerable. You are *both* feeling scared and insecure about the future. When you can both voice your pain and fears honestly, you allow yourselves to be seen and supported, thereby strengthening your relationship and endurance.

PATIENT PERSPECTIVE: JORGE-ARMANDO D., HIV

HIV came into my life at a young age, when it felt like life was just beginning. I was starting to heal my childhood traumas as I navigated adult life, trying to accept who I was. It was difficult to accept my sexual identity, coming from a Latino culture that taught me that being gay was wrong and shameful. For me, college was a safe place. It was a place where I learned to challenge what I didn't agree with, a place that allowed me to begin to love and accept myself. However, at 21 years old, HIV entered my life, and my life changed forever.

I read somewhere the definition of endurance: "Endurance is the virtue exhibited by someone who characteristically puts up with adversity, pain, discomfort, hardship, or suffering in a way that allows them to maintain their poise." I agree. I used to believe that HIV robbed me of my happiness and so many opportunities; it nearly destroyed me at such a young age. However, in my darkest and most lonely moments, I learned to rebuild, forgive, and heal. It has taken me over twenty years to get here, but after hardship, suffering, and pain, I stand with such inner beauty and poise. In that way, HIV freed me and taught me and has given me a voice and platform larger than life itself.

ENDURE PATIENTLY

If you were to Google the word "endure," this is what you'd find:

> *v.* (1) suffer something painful or difficult patiently; (2) remain in existence, last.

This is where the "patience" of the Patient's Journey becomes so important. In this difficult, painful experience of disease, to *endure* means to navigate the road patiently. And to *endure* also means to remain and last. Your outcome as a patient will be stronger if you look for ways to optimize your life in the long haul. Don't get mired in thoughts about death. *Look to last*, in the best, most positive way you can.

As you do so, you build enormous resilience and inner strength. In fact, when endurance is used in the context of exercise, it means "the ability of an organism to exert itself and remain active for a long period of time, as well as its ability to resist, withstand, recover from and have immunity to trauma, wounds or fatigue."* *Resist. Withstand. Recover from. Have IMMUNITY to trauma, wounds, or fatigue.* Those are powerful words!

---

* "Endurance," Wikipedia, accessed March 16, 2023, https://en.wikipedia.org/wiki/Endurance.

By pushing through when you are at your weakest, you are building untold strength. That inner strength and resilience will serve you for the rest of your life—as long as you endure.

STAGE 6 OF THE PATIENT'S JOURNEY: ENDURANCE

- *Common emotions: periodic fatigue or frustration at all the necessary trial and error, eventual increase in positivity and energy, a mix between resolve and resignation.*

- *Common pitfalls: neglecting to care for the people in your orbit, not communicating with family or work supervisors about necessary shifts in the division of labor, trying to do too many of the things you used to do, putting off necessary effort toward healing, or failing to enlist needed help.*

- *Your best next step: Say "no" when you need to, be proactive in your communication, express gratitude, and be strategic about crafting your best new normal! Whatever energy you have in you—use it. Expect this stage to feel like a slog and continue to persevere.*

CHAPTER 8

Optimize Your Relationships

CONNECTING AND EVOLVING WITH YOUR PEOPLE

"Alone, we can do so little. Together, we can do so much."

— Helen Keller

You're learning your "new normal" on this Patient's Journey: your new body, your new routine, your new capabilities, new boundaries, and new medications.

But one of the most significant areas to experience the ripple effect of your disease is in your relationships. All the people around you are trying to learn *their* "new normal," too. And because of that, your relational dynamics may shift.

That shift *can* be a good thing. Anyone who engages in the Patient's Journey will grow in empathy and resilience, which are profound gifts. Many relationships strengthen through this Journey—but not all. The stress of disease is also not something to underestimate. And because of that, one entire chapter of the Patient's Journey is devoted to the intentional communication that's required to Optimize Your Relationships.

For everyone involved in this Patient's Journey, your greatest tools for connection will be transparency, vulnerability, openness, and loving feedback. When you lean toward each other in intentional ways, relationships can become a source of strength—rather than stress—to propel you all toward greater wholeness.

Sickness can be a source of huge stress on relationships, causing strain. But when you lean toward each other in intentional ways, relationships can become a source of strength to propel you and your loved ones toward greater wholeness.

THE NEW NORMAL

My daughter became my wheelchair pusher. My dad became my cheerleader. My aunt became my chief researcher. When my mom visited, she did every house chore known to humankind, and when my sister came, she listened. All of them: taking on new roles, as I took on the role of patient.

Before I got so sick, I used to walk Stephanie to school. Her kindergarten was just a few blocks from our place and across a busy street. In my pre-MS life, I always made Steph hold my hand. I never let her cross that busy street alone.

After MS, it was different. I was home in a wheelchair, but I still wanted to take her to school. I wanted to be her mom and do the things that were "normal." So, we developed a new routine. I made Steph her toast, using a little gripping tool to pull items out of the cupboard. (I MADE THE TOAST.) At 7:45 a.m., Stephanie opened the door and held it for me while I rolled my wheelchair out. She shut the door behind me, and I reached up to lock it. Then, my six-year-old pushed my wheelchair down the street.

When Steph pushed me to the large intersection where we had to cross the street, I raised my voice to be heard above the traffic noise. "Wait until it turns green, honey!" When the light changed, I called, "Okay sweetie, we can go now!" My brave little daughter pushed me forward and I used my one good arm to help us along across the street. Her head barely came up over the back of the wheelchair. But we'd make our way across.

We got to the school campus, and she kissed me goodbye, then scampered off to her classroom. I wheeled myself around and began struggling my way back home. I felt so proud of both of us—me, for basically being Rocky and getting my girl to school on time—and her, for being the sweetest, bravest, strongest little six-year-old I knew. Both of us were figuring out our new normal, which included figuring out new capabilities.

My dad's role in my life had always been that of provider, caretaker, the guy who could fix things. (Or at least find someone else to fix things!) But when I got sick, he couldn't fix me. He could take me to appointments, he could protect me from asshole doctors—but there was nothing he could actually do to "fix" his daughter, and that was incredibly hard for him. As we navigated our relationship in the context of this new normal, his role shifted. He became my motivator. He was my encourager. He was the one who gave me a kick in the ass when I needed it to keep on trying.

My aunt Melinda took on the role of being one of my main care partners. She was a nurse and became my chief researcher. Even before I got diagnosed, it was Melinda who had figured out that I probably had MS, from all the reading she had done. And after my diagnosis, she continued to take the lead on learning about the disease and researching potential advances in MS.

She also became my advocate. There was one night when I was still in the hospital, fighting off yet another MS relapse, and they had given me a strong mix of medications. Melinda came in and recognized that I was out of it. *Really* out of it. She checked the monitors and could see that my respiratory rate was extremely low. Melinda went out into the hall and waved down the healthcare team. "She's allergic to a bunch of medications," she said. "I don't know what you guys have her on, but she's not doing well."

One of the nurses said, "We gave her something to help her sleep. She's on such a high dose of steroids, it's almost impossible to fall asleep."

"Well, it's too much," Melinda said. "Have you seen her respiratory rate? You guys need to get in here!"

And then the healthcare team collectively had an "Oh shit" moment.

Before I knew it, I was on a nasal cannula and they were pumping in oxygen. I don't even remember that night because I was so out of it—Melinda had to tell me what happened later.

Melinda's not a confrontational person. She's not a clinical nurse either; she's an occupational nurse. But my vulnerability as Patient called up her strength as Advocate. She went out there and said, "I need you to come in right now and see this." And she continued to advocate for me throughout my Patient's Journey. She also made herself an expert about my medications and available healthcare choices.

This is the strange evolution that happens to the people around you as you travel this Patient's Journey: your loved ones start learning new skills. They discover abilities they didn't know they had. Everyone starts realizing they can handle more than they thought they could. They take on new roles. They become passionate advocates about issues that weren't even on their radar a year ago. And as you and your loved ones evolve personally, your relationships evolve, too. There's work to be done to navigate these relationships successfully. Relationships are hard in the best of times, but sickness can make them much harder. You're grumpy, you don't feel well, you're tired, you're crabby. There are gross things to deal with: bodily functions and clean up and unpleasant symptoms. And your people are worried, they're stressed, and they're *also* tired; they feel burdened with fear and heightened responsibility. No one is functioning at their best.

That's why communication is vital, and vulnerability is needed. Through intentional communication, you can strengthen your relationships on this journey, rather than watch them suffer. You can evolve together into a much stronger team.

The Patient's Journey prompts an evolution for patients, care partners, and everyone touched by the disease; it also causes relationships to evolve. The strategies you hone when optimizing relationships will be ones you use throughout the different seasons of your illness and life.

But, let's not sugarcoat it. Disease is fucking hard for everyone involved. Let's start by acknowledging the ways sickness can generate stress on relationships.

YES, DISEASE CAN IMPAIR CONNECTION

I'm going to give you the bad news first. (But this isn't the end of the story, so keep reading.) Disease *can* impair connection. That may be obvious by now.

The physical parts of disease pose plenty of hurdles. You go from being a healthy person to being someone who struggles to walk, or move, or get out of bed, or give yourself treatment. The ripple effects of that are immediate. You can't walk around an amusement park with your friends. You can't run the Jingle Bell 5k with your work colleagues. You're not able to chaperone your kid's field trip to the zoo. Some people with seizure disorders can no longer drive their car, so now they're housebound. If you have any form of metastatic cancer, you tend to get told it's not *if* you die but *when* you die, and that fact can add huge intensity to your relational connections. The path of least resistance might be to simply avoid connection altogether, because whatever relationship you form is understood to have an expiration date.

I know of children who have a genetic condition that causes them to develop blindness, and their parents must grapple with their child not being able to visually connect with them anymore. Amputations are a reality for some patients, such as survivors of meningococcal meningitis or people with uncontrolled diabetes; you may not be able to pick up your loved one from work or lift a child out of its crib when the necessary limbs are missing. Some patients with eczema feel barriers in cuddling their young children, due to the roughness of their skin. Disease is no joke. These are incredibly challenging realities to live with and can easily pose difficulties for relational connection.

Physical intimacy is its own category of challenge and also a huge loss for many patients. I've seen relationships end because of this particular loss. Even when sex is still physically possible, many medications have side effects that make physical intimacy hard. Certain meds can impact libido, cause sleepiness, or prompt weight gain or other physical changes that weaken your self-esteem. And let's not forget, the combination of your disease and your medication might just make you feel extremely unsexy. That reality can create huge difficulties for people in a romantic partnership.

It's not just physical connection that disease can mess with—the bigger challenge, often, is emotional.

It's not just physical connection that disease can mess with—the bigger challenge, often, is emotional. Internally, patients are going through that identity earthquake. Many of your core values and the way you've shown up for the majority of your life has been completely upended by the nature of your diagnosis. It's hard enough to keep yourself together and tap into your new normal, let alone show up in your personal relationships with perfect emotional equilibrium. You have self-doubt, you're worried, you feel insecure, and you struggle with questions like, "Is my partner staying with me out of pity? Have I ruined my family's life? Am I even worth being loved?" There are enormous emotional roadblocks, which make it hard to simply flip the switch to physically connect during "sexy time."

The combination of physical *and* emotional challenges can make things tough for care partners as well. If their loved one says something like, "I have a headache today," or, "I'm not up for it," that doesn't necessarily indicate the patient's emotional withdrawal—

it may be a totally legitimate physical roadblock, or the patient's own emotional struggle. But that's not necessarily how the care partner may experience it. They might think, "Oh, they just don't like me anymore." Usually, that's not the case at all! But because physical withdrawal can *look* like emotional withdrawal and is sometimes mistaken for it, you must both address the situation openly.

Here's the good news though: work-arounds exist. They start with open communication.

WORK-AROUNDS

Therein lies the best way forward: if you *can* be open and vulnerable—if you *can* be honest about what you're dealing with—often, profound solutions can come. There's a work-around for almost every kind of connection challenge out there.

Consider the physical intimacy piece. Option 1: you stay silent about not wanting intimacy or not being able to have sex. You don't bring up that symptom with your doctor. It becomes the Big Monster in your relationship. You start to check out. You stop emotionally connecting. The relationship becomes burdened by the stress of your disease, compounded by the lack of connection on all fronts.

That's not a great option.

Option 2: you initiate the conversation. Granted, that's not easy. You let your partner know why or how it's hard to be physically intimate. You talk about the symptoms with your doctor and see if any help is available. Then, you start brainstorming work-arounds with your partner.

There are ways to enjoy intimacy that might simply require a more unconventional approach. I don't want to get too kinky on anyone, but many disabled people avail themselves of tools. I'm not talking about hammers and wrenches—I'm talking about sexy tools. Even conservative disabled people who thought they would never "go there" find new possibilities for their intimacy through the use of sex toys like vibrators and dildos. (Did I really just go there? Yes, I did. You're welcome.)

I'll never forget one patient who shared with a counseling group. Her advice was candid: "Think Nike," she said. "You've just got to *do it*. You've got to get back on the horse and ride." Of course, I loved her analogy. She went on to explain: "I just had to start having sex again. I didn't even like it at first, but I just knew that I had to do it and make it happen. In my mind, I had to get it over with. But then it became, 'Oh, hey ... We like this! It's a little bit different, but this is good!'"

Now is the time to get creative looking into devices or positions you may not have felt comfortable exploring before. Where there's a will, there's a way! And here's the silver lining: if you can push through these new layers of vulnerability and navigate these intimacy challenges with your partner, you will come out the other side much more deeply connected.

Creative work-arounds exist, but if you hope to find them, you must be brave enough to open the conversation.

I do want to acknowledge that the physical intimacy piece can be a roller coaster, with a lot of ups and downs. There may be times when your physical symptoms are such that you simply can't imagine having sex, and no amount of "just do it" slogans could get you to make things hot in the sack. But don't buy into the lie that you're only intimate if you have sex. "Intimacy" comes in more forms than merely physical. The intimacy you cultivate with your partner is also emotional, intellectual, and spiritual—it's all the close, vulnerable ways you connect to your special person that make the relationship different than the one you share with someone like your sibling.

Lean into those other forms of intimacy during the times when your physical symptoms make sex feel impossible. What are other ways you can still cultivate and harbor intimacy? The most vital investment in your intimacy will come via open, honest conversation— whether that's about the challenges of physical intimacy, how you're *really* feeling, the spiritual realizations you're having, or a new mental reframe that's been helpful. Vulnerability and honesty will help keep your intimate connection alive, even during times when physical intimacy is impossible.

If you're struggling to overcome the emotional connection barrier, counseling can be helpful. Many organizations offer subsidized or free counseling. There are also many forums to connect online with other patients who might be dealing with similar challenges.

But remember the most important strategies that we've already discussed in this book, those that arise out of your own head and heart: The determination to choose hope and positivity. The courage to be honest. The willingness to be vulnerable. Whether you're a patient or caregiver, as much as possible, stay connected to the hobbies and things that make you "you." Those pastimes will help you remember that you're not just a person who goes to the hospital a lot—you are a loving, interesting, desirable, amazing person.

Yes, disease can be isolating. But at some point, you're going to need to take a big step forward and decide to go back to the land of the living. Become a joiner again and *get back at it*—whether that means choosing to "just do it" in the bedroom, or risking a vulnerable conversation, or showing up to your kid's soccer game in a wheelchair, or cuddling your children even though you feel lousy. You can do this on your terms when the time is right. The majority of people living with tough medical conditions become very choosy about who they're connecting to, and then they go all in with those relationships. That's appropriate. You can be strategic about the when and the how and the who.

But then, *with* those close relationships, focus on pushing through the challenges to deeper connection. Be honest with them, because that will help build your connection back from some of the strain your disease may have created. In problem solving together and finding new, creative ways to connect, you'll discover a level of closeness that you may not have ever experienced before.

On that note, let's examine the silver lining.

DISEASE CAN ALSO HELP FORGE STRONGER CONNECTIONS

Here's the good news: you can actually come away with *stronger* connections because of your disease. I developed a much deeper connection to my special people as a result of my MS shining a bright light on my own mortality. It crystallized for me how I most want to spend my time.

The most significant relationship in my life where that connection deepened was with my daughter. We had an *intense* experience navigating my MS together from the time that she was young, but that has made the two of us incredibly close. Other than me, Stephanie is more in tune with the little nuances of my health than anyone else.

She'll spot a symptom in me before anyone else sees it. She and I have a closeness and safety to be honest in our relationship that has been forged through us navigating this disease together.

There is a "watch out" here though, because it can be easy to create codependency in the patient/caregiver relationship. As close as Stephanie and I are, I wouldn't ever want her to live by me just so she could take care of me. If she lives near me because she also likes the town, and the schools for her daughter, and the community— then, that's wonderful. But I want her to feel the freedom for her own life to move forward. Your special people need to be able to go where *they* need to be. If they don't have that freedom, the relationship can easily become brittle because of resentment and a sense of being trapped.

It can be easy to create codependency in the patient/caregiver relationship, which can lead to resentment. Your loved ones need freedom for their lives to move forward.

The best possible set up for relationships to forge a deeper bond is for both the patient and care partner to meet these traumas head on, have healing conversations, and make sure everyone is moving forward on this Journey, to the best of their abilities.

It's true that disease can be hard on connection, but when you tackle something really hard and intense with another person— especially if it's something most people don't experience—that creates a special, powerful, unique bond.

I mentioned that I had seen many relationships end because of the strain on connection created by disease. Hopefully, this book can help couples dealing with the same challenges to maintain and strengthen their mutual commitment instead of giving up on one another. I've also seen just as many relationships forge a *deeper* connection. The couples that stay together often seem to have an extra special layer of "life's purpose" folded into their relationship. On the one hand, they look toward the future and consider how the experience of navigating disease might make them stronger. They ask questions like, "How can we let this deepen our empathy for others? How might this make us more available to serve or care for people, down the road? How can we find hope in the thought that these experiences will not go to waste?" By focusing on the shared purpose they might uncover in the future, they strengthen their own connection.

And it's also helpful when couples focus on the *now*. With your "special glasses" on, the present becomes that much more precious and meaningful, because you're aware that every moment counts. You stop thinking so much about "when the kids move out," or "when we retire," or "when we have the money"—because you can't wait! Every minute of every day offers the chance to achieve your "together" goals and enjoy a deep, connected, fun life.

Enduring disease alongside your loved ones can also help you grow emotionally in profound ways—another gift. I can think of a couple I met some years ago. The husband was a police officer who was so preoccupied with his line of duty, he tried to avoid letting any emotions "cloud" his judgment. He viewed himself as a machine that needed to function. Then, his wife got cancer, which caused her to go blind. She ultimately passed away, but before she did, they spent years working through her cancer together. The experience completely transformed her husband, and he became a much more emotive person. He became a great "teen dad" to his adolescent girls, patiently walking alongside them through their hormonal changes and relationship dramas. He also excelled professionally and got promoted. It turns out he *didn't* need to function as a machine to be a great cop. Although the loss of his wife was shattering, their journey through her disease transformed him into someone who cherished the little things in life and who understood that he, too, was only human.

Another couple had to push hard to forge a deeper connection and almost didn't manage it. But once they opened the doors of honesty and vulnerability, everything changed. Henry was diagnosed with a severe and aggressive form of rheumatoid arthritis (RA). He had already been slightly "curmudgeonly"—he was a hard-working introvert who tended to keep to himself. The diagnosis intensified his tendency to turn inward. It also meant he wasn't able to do Kung Fu anymore, which had been one of his passions. He didn't have any of the tools or skills to communicate transparently about what he was experiencing. And as a result, his relationship with his wife, Shannon, began to fall apart.

They were on the brink of divorce when I met him through a meeting hosted by Snow Companies. Henry got connected with us because he had elected to be one of the first patients to take a newly FDA-approved drug for his type of RA, and we were filming stories about patients' journeys. I met him and Shannon on a Thursday night. Shannon was clearly nervous, talking for the both of them. You could see she was eager to be liked. He, on the other hand, remained emotionally closed and didn't give off any warm vibes. I know now, he was scared.

I knew I wanted to help him and provide a safe space for him to process. Over the next four days, we walked patients and their care partners through a storytelling workshop, doing activities to help them find their voice, share their story, and dig deep. I could *see* Henry's shell cracking. I was the facilitator that weekend and tailored a lot of my information and comments toward Henry in an effort to help. On Thursday, he was aloof and cold. On Friday, he had opened up a bit. Then, on Saturday, there was a breakthrough. He cried when he was writing his story.

On Sunday, the group of twenty patients and care partners gathered to share the first iteration of their stories. Before anyone got started, Shannon jumped out of her seat and said, "This is the best weekend ever! Henry did *so* good. And last night, we really connected; we had SEX!" Henry turned about ten shades of red. "He's never talked to me about his disease," Shannon continued. "He's never shared anything about what it's been like for him, but now I understand. And we feel more connected than we ever have—he's never made me feel this way."

As they were leaving the workshop that weekend, they both pulled me aside. "Thank you for saving our marriage," Henry said.

He went on to be the keynote speaker at an event for a huge biotech company with close to a thousand people in the audience. The drug had been helping his RA, but Henry was transformed for reasons beyond that. He had a complete attitude change—he *exuded* positivity. There was such a transformation, with him being connected to his wife again and connecting to his own story. He came on stage in his Kung Fu outfit and did a martial arts move as he entered. Then, he opened up and shared with everyone the powerful personal narrative that had been so huge in helping him reconnect with Shannon.

At the end of his speech, Shannon got up and took the mic. "I just want to say one thing today," she said. "This experience of Henry telling his story has saved our marriage. And I just want to thank all of you for being part of it."

When Shannon and Henry got vulnerable and honest with each other, they were able to take a critical step forward. I think a big reason for that was because Henry realized the true value of connection. That was what helped them get unstuck.

The same is true for you. If you can't recognize the value of authentically connecting with the people around you, it will be difficult to move your life forward. Optimizing your relationships *is part of your healing process*. Believe that! Disease can help you forge deeper, stronger, more meaningful connections with the people you love—provided you have the courage to be vulnerable and share openly with them.

Disease can help you forge stronger connections with the people you love—provided you have the courage to be vulnerable and share openly with them.

And keep in mind that, especially for anyone with a chronic illness, impediments to connection will ebb and flow over the course of a lifetime. Expect to *continue* being vulnerable and honest with each other; just because you solved an issue once doesn't mean it's not going to come up again.

It's in the context of these relationships that you'll find, once again, what fills up your cup. These healthy relationships will give to you and enable you to give to others. That experience will start to make you feel whole again.

COMMUNICATING ABOUT YOUR ILLNESS

But let's look beyond care partners now. There are *many* people who will be in your orbit. In fact, you need a team around you. Recruiting that team can be hard, though, especially if you're feeling hesitant to open up about your illness on a larger scale.

A lot of patients decide not to disclose. Some are afraid of losing their job. Or maybe they're simply afraid of judgment and what other people might think or say. This is understandable, but nine times out of ten, you're going to be better off simply being transparent about what's going on.

Some patients don't want to alert their employers to their illness. They may fear they'd lose their job, that there would be talk behind their back, or that they would be treated differently. And those fears are not completely unfounded, though there are laws in place to protect people with diseases in the workplace. Still, I highly recommend you do share about your illness. If you don't tell, there are no reasonable accommodations to make your life easier, and you'll be held to the exact same standards and performance levels as you were pre-diagnosis.

Few people—especially when they're still early in the Diagnosis phase—can keep performing at their previous level when they're suffering. If your employer is in the dark about your illness, they'll assume you're simply becoming a subpar employee: "What happened to So-and-So? They're really off their game lately. Seeing some major performance issues." You may get put on a Performance Improvement Plan, and before you know it, if you want to save your job, you'll *have* to fess up about your illness. Better to just do it earlier and save yourself from weeks or months of bad press and critical assumptions. Not only will people typically respond with empathy and understanding, but you'll also set yourself up to gather that necessary team around you. Many coworkers will be eager to help you in whatever way they can.

There's still the matter of *how* though. *How* are you going to tell your employer? And what the hell are you going to say to your parents? To your kids? To your extended family, your friends, and your team members? Usually, this communication needs to happen right away—often much earlier than you'd prefer. Before you've even fully comprehended what's going on in your body, you need to figure out what you're going to tell other people—and in some cases, what you're *not* going to tell them.

You need to figure out what you're going to tell other people about your illness—and in some cases, what you're *not* going to tell them. You also need to make a plan about *how*.

Me, I told everybody. I didn't bother filtering much out, either. But that's an individual choice, and I completely respect people who choose to disclose less. Regardless of where you fall on that spectrum, you need to make some communication decisions:

- *Who* are you going to tell?
- *What* are you going to say about your illness? And how might you change the messaging, depending on who you're telling?

- *How* are you going to say it? Are you going to do a mass post on Facebook or CaringBridge? A mass text to a curated list of people? Phone calls? In-person meetings? Or a combination of all of the above?
- *When* are you going to communicate about this? You might elect to share with some key people immediately but put off informing your employer for a little longer.

Answering these questions should be the basis of your communication strategy and plan. This can be uncomfortable, but once the news is out, the help can start rolling in.

Your Emotional Support Team

Let's talk about some of the other people you need on your support team. I'm not talking about your medical and financial support team yet—your therapists, specialists, social workers, legal helpers, and all the rest. We'll get to them in the next chapter. But one of the linchpins in your ability to endure this illness for the long haul is building up a strong *emotional* support team. You need these people—and they need you. Here are some of the main people you need on your team, along with some recommendations for how you can nurture your relationship with them:

- **Like-minded patients:** It's helpful to be able to connect with other people who have the same disease as you. In fact, those may become some of the most important people on your team. With all that said, though, make sure the patients you connect with are similarly motivated to progress on their Patient's Journey and aren't keeping themselves stuck in a pity party. I didn't want to be "just" the MS patient, and I didn't want to spend time with people who were defining themselves in terms of their disease. I wanted to connect with others who knew we were *more* than the sum of our symptoms and could spur each other toward hope and wholeness. Sometimes you can find these other patients through advocacy organizations; the internet is also an incredible resource to seek out these connections. For many conditions, life science companies are running various kinds of patient connection programs, many of which are managed by Snow Companies.

- **Friends that "get it":** It's a huge gift to have a group of friends that won't feel compelled to give you advice or instruction, or offer dumb clichés. The best sorts of friends are the ones who can handle your TMI, will talk to you about things other than being sick, can remind you of who you are, can make you laugh, won't feel uncomfortable with your tears, and don't mind helping out in little ways. I had a core group of four friends, and I was able to tell them things I couldn't tell anyone else on this list.

- **Your kids:** (If you've got them.) Many people try to hide their condition from their kids, or at least mask the pain of it. I always tell people, "Share at an age-appropriate level. You can give your kids a real gift by being transparent with them." I tried to be reassuring with Stephanie when she felt afraid or worried for

me, but we also had frank discussions about my limitations, even when she was quite young. She knew exactly
what I could and couldn't do. In learning about that,
she grew up with a lot of empathy for other people. I
shared about how she became my wheelchair docent:
she'd hold open the doors and call out, "Look out! My
mom's coming through!" When she was ten, long after
I had regained my ability to walk, Stephanie saw a man
in a wheelchair struggling to get through a door. She
ran and held the door open for him. When he thanked
her and told her what a nice young lady she was, she
said, "Well, I know about this, because my mom's in a
wheelchair sometimes, too." That was a beautiful conclusion to many frustrating non-walking years: my
daughter had become an expert in seeing and caring
for other people.

- **Other family members:** You need your family—but
you also need your family to follow your rules of
engagement. Plenty of family members can be a drain
on your energy. Keep those engagements rare and
short. However, those family members who can support you in the mission you've set for yourself and
march to the beat of your drum—hold them close.

- **Spiritual community:** Spirituality means different
things to different people, but let me tell you—I see
patients benefiting profoundly when they have a spiritual connection to prayer or meditation, can identify
their life's purpose, and sense there's a larger plan they
can find hope in. Some people find a spiritual

community in yoga; other people find this connection in a more traditional church setting. These groups of people can help support you in both practical and intangible ways—bringing you meals, giving your kids rides, doing your laundry … And also praying for you, texting you encouragement, or sending you a beautiful song to listen to. This spiritual community is important for a lot of patients to have on their team.

PATIENT PERSPECTIVE: RICK S., EPILEPSY

I remember when someone showed me how much I truly mattered. It was during my Patient Ambassador meeting in 2007. Listening to other patients' stories, I didn't feel that my story was important or that I could have the impact the other Ambassadors had on me. Honestly, I left the room looking for someplace to hide until we went back to the hotel, before they could all discover what a phony I was. I was desperate to find a way out.

Brenda noticed my absence almost immediately and came looking for me. She found me in the lobby; I was trembling, crying, and confused about what I could offer anyone. She put her arm around me and told me she strongly believed I had the power to make an impact. She held me and let me cry a little, then she told me to come back to the conference room when I was ready. During this time, I later found out, she spoke to another attendee and asked him to provide support and encouragement to me. That person became one of my closest friends. I've never felt so much love and acceptance for my epilepsy, which has been the one thing that always made me feel like an outsider.

Get Them Off Your Team

Part of optimizing your team also involves kicking certain people *off* your team. To make this easy for you, I'm going to call out some of the negative people who don't deserve a place in your orbit. Boundary the hell out of these folks:

- **Snake oil salesmen:** The healthcare and self-care industries are enormous, and it is *full* of wooden charlatans who want to try to sell you the "miracle cure." Unfortunately, there are also a lot of well-meaning people who buy into those false claims and come to you with elated promises that some bizarre remedy will cure you. I subscribe to hope but *not* to false hope, and these snake oil salesmen are trying to sell you a bill of goods. If you want to try them, fine—most of them won't hurt. (Though some could!) You need to be careful, with both your hopes and the money you consider spending. Also, remember that even the best therapy is only *one* piece of the pie as far as your healing goes. Your mindset, healthcare team, and all the other modalities to strengthen your body also really matter. So, if anyone comes to you and says, "All you need to do is [this miracle cure] and you'll get better! The pharmaceutical industry and your doctor don't want you to know about it, but it works!"—run in the other direction.

- **Pity-me patients:** Avoid the patients who are keen to tell you that everything is a piece of shit. These negative people will pull you down! They haven't gotten the

memo that this isn't the way to live. Their coping mechanism is to make you miserable because *they're* miserable. Yikes.

- **Bad healthcare professionals:** I alluded to this already,
but listen. If they don't listen, or validate you; if they
don't believe you; if they don't spend time with you; if
they don't order the tests you think you need—you
don't want them around!

- **Friends who see you in terms of your limits:** A lot of
people just don't know what to do with sickies. They're
not necessarily bad actors, but they put limiting boundaries on you. I'm talking about friends who stop including you because they assume you can't do something,
or people that don't know how to talk to you about
anything other than your illness. I used to let those
people hurt my feelings and cause me to feel insecure,
but as I got more confident, I realized I didn't want to
be around those people anyway. Life is too short for
people who pull you down instead of lift you up. As
much as you can, graciously look to step away from
those people.

- **People who say dumb things:** You know what I'm talking about. These are the people that attempt to empathize in insensitive ways: "Oh, I know exactly how you
feel. When I get sick, all I want to do is lay on the couch
and binge TV." Or they want to fix you somehow.
Some people feel like they need to give you some great
nugget of wisdom that will change your mindset. For
some of those people, you can simply ice them out and

ghost them. Or, for people that you can't do that with, reeducate them. Say, "I know you're trying to be helpful, but it's actually not helpful. Let me tell you why." Either graciously leave or meet it head on.

WHAT IF I'M ALONE?

Some patients reading this might see the words "emotional support team" and think, "Yeah, right." Post-pandemic, America is lonelier than it's ever been, a trend some researchers have labeled an epidemic.* Many people feel isolated, and you might be in a spot where you *don't* have a care partner that can step up in these different ways. Maybe you don't see a larger network of communities that you can tap into. For whatever reason: you're alone.

For all the patients that feel this way—I want to issue you a challenge. There is *somebody* that cares for you. It might be the Sunday school teacher at your church that you only see a couple times a year. It might be your next-door neighbor that you think is too busy with their own family. It might be a colleague that you used to work with that you haven't seen in a while. But I'm telling you, those people are out there. You might even have a name in your mind right now.

In my experience being a patient, I have found that the phrase "I need help" tends to bring out the best in human nature. People *want* to be helpful. They want to be utilized. When you ask for

---

* Cashin, Ali. "Loneliness in America: How the Pandemic Has Deepened an Epidemic of Loneliness and What We Can Do About It." Making Caring Common Project. February 9, 2021. https://mcc.gse.harvard.edu/reports/loneliness-in-america.

help, what's the worst response you might realistically get? People could say "no." Big deal. That won't leave you any worse off than if you hadn't asked. In most cases, you'll get a "yes," as long as whatever you're asking for is reasonable. It's worth asking either way.

If you feel like you have no one to provide you with emotional support, please: overcome the fear of not wanting to bother people. We so often think, "I don't want to ask that person and burden them ... " But there is *somebody* out there who would be honored if you asked for their help.

That doesn't mean you ask that person to sit on the phone with Social Security for ten hours—at least, not at your first get together. But there are people who would love to connect with you. As you do, the relationship will evolve, and they may become someone who *would* sit on the phone that long on your behalf. Or mow your lawn, or get your groceries, or whatever else you might need. Your people are out there. They just need a nudge.

The worst thing you can do as a patient is to choose to believe that you are permanently and unavoidably alone. If you live in that mindset, you will paralyze your ability to move forward on this journey.

The worst thing you can do as a patient is to choose to believe that you are permanently and unavoidably alone. There is *somebody* who cares for you.

Reach out. Look up a patient support group. Text an old friend you haven't talked to in a while. Open up a little when your neighbor asks how you're doing. Try out your local church. Whatever this looks like for you—evolve into a new normal where people are allowed to care for you.

MESSAGE TO CARE PARTNERS: YOUR RELATIONSHIPS

Heads up care partners: you have some responsibilities in this phase, too. As you navigate relationships in your own version of the Patient's Journey, you need to proactively communicate and develop your own emotional support team.

Many people have walked in your shoes before you, and they have tips and strategies that they've used with their own loved ones. They've found work-arounds; they've discovered things that have worked. Find those people! They will be safe for you to vent to, which is something you desperately need. There will be times when you need to say, "I'm so *over* this today. I had no idea how hard it would be. I hate what's happened." You need to be able to talk about that with someone—but *not* the patient you're caring for. As much as you two will want to be open and vulnerable with each other, there's a difference between being thoughtfully honest and venting in such a way that you cause lasting damage. You *do* need to vent to someone—but not your loved one fighting illness.

Also, communicate with your loved one about what your "lanes" are. Caregiving is straightforward enough when it's just about helping out in the bathroom or preparing the food. But what about doctors' appointments? Who's going to do the bulk of the communication? Who's going to ask the questions? These are points that would be helpful to talk about ahead of time. Be really clear about what the patient will do, versus what you do.

Your presence will always be valuable as a second set of ears, but your role will fluctuate beyond that. If your loved one is in an acute part of their journey, they may not have the energy to make the phone calls and set up appointments. In those times, you may have to step up as a stronger advocate, like Melinda was for me. Turn up the heat when it needs to be turned up.

Other times, the patient might feel more ready to advocate for themselves and it's appropriate for you to let them lead.

All of these shifts will be best navigated with clear communication. Say back to your loved one, "This is what I'm hearing you say. Am I understanding this correctly? Am I tracking?" You want to avoid making assumptions about what they want. Instead, just ask. If at all possible, don't try to fill in the blanks by yourself. Frequent, regular communication will be your best tool to maintain the health of your relationship.

EVOLVING ROLES

Remember the gifts we talked about in Chapter 6? Disease comes with a heavy set of burdens, but it also comes with impossibly beautiful gifts. And the beauty of being human is that we are interconnected. A Patient's Journey affects *many* people. As the patient evolves, their loved ones must evolve, too. That means the burdens are shared—and so are the gifts.

Watch your people and marvel as you navigate this journey together. You'll be amazed as you view them through the lenses of your special glasses!

On the other side of your children's emotional messiness, you will witness them arriving at deeper empathy, compassion, and responsibility. On the other side of the conflicts and tensions with your care partner, you will be amazed at the depth, freedom, and connection you two discover. On the other side of struggle, you will see the people in your orbit step up in kindness, strength, advocacy, expertise, and resilience. *If* you engage in the hard conversations. *If* you choose to be vulnerable. *If* you open the door to face the hard questions. *If* you push past points of tension to seek out creative work-arounds. It's this brave act of opening yourself up that brings you and your loved ones closer. And that's the gift of the new normal.

STAGE 7 OF THE PATIENT'S JOURNEY: OPTIMIZE YOUR RELATIONSHIPS

- *Common emotions: impatience or frustration with your loved ones; gratitude for what they are doing or trying to do; guilt for not living up to your own expectations.*
- *Common pitfalls: Trying to go it alone. Lack of clarity about what you need, what you want, and what you can and cannot do. And even if there's clarity about your needs, there can still often be a lack of communication.*
- *Your best next step: Let go of shame and embarrassment. Find your voice and share your needs. Focus on building a team.*

CHAPTER 9

Optimize Your Care

LEARN TO SELF-ADVOCATE TO GET THE KNOWLEDGE YOU NEED

"What we find changes who we become."

— Peter Morville

*L*earning. That's a huge element of what you're doing throughout the long Endurance phase. You're learning what routines work best, what processes work best, where you need to set boundaries, what needs to be communicated, and so on. You're optimizing, through trial and error.

Optimizing your care requires that you learn an enormous wealth of *information* about your disease and everything related to it. In fact, you need cutting-edge information—not just about the drugs you need to take or the therapies you need. You need information about how to talk to your family about this, how to manage your symptoms, how to delay the recurrence of the disease, what nonmedical modalities will actually help you, how to live on a reduced income, how to avail yourself of legal help when needed, how to navigate advanced directives, and so on.

Unfortunately, even though you need this information, there's no specialty store of information tailored to your specific body, disease, and circumstances, where it's all gathered in one place. That's why, in the Optimize Your Care stage, you need to aggressively self-advocate. You need to actively seek out information to optimize your healthcare plan. Earlier in your Patient's Journey, you were learning like crazy—but you were mostly *receiving* information. You were *comprehending*. You were doing your best to *absorb* it all. In other words, the information was largely being presented *to you* as a recipient, and you were doing your best just to take it all in.

You're doing something different in this stage. You are *seeking it out*. You are *pursuing* it. You are *hunting it down*. You are now taking on the role of a proactive, engaged patient, looking to learn as much as possible about what will help you.

If you think this sounds like it requires energy, you're right. If you think it sounds like you might even need to be aggressive—you're right. You need both energy and aggressiveness to optimize your care, and when you can't muster them, you need to deputize your care partner to wield them for you. And here's why:

You don't get what you don't ask for. Being a badass sickie means you have to ruthlessly advocate for yourself to get the information and medicine you need.

Be a badass sickie: ruthlessly advocate for yourself to get the information and medicine you need. You don't get what you don't ask for.

In my own Patient's Journey, I needed a push to get me to level up to the kind of self-advocacy I deserved. But once I went there, I didn't stop. The rewards of advocating for myself in the pursuit of information far outweighed the risks.

"YOU NEED TO TALK TO ME."

Two and a half years after getting diagnosed, things were still not great, but they had improved. I'd been taking Betaseron for a year and a half, which had helped me improve. I was even walking again. I needed to use a cane—but I was on my feet. Thank you, science; thank you, endless hours of physical therapy; and thank you, positive attitude!

The bad news: I still understood very little about my actual disease. The lack of patient information at that time was staggering—MS was basically a footnote in a 1956 medical journal.

On top of that, taking my drug was a giant pain in my ass—and I mean that literally. I had to give myself injections every other day. The process involved sticking a tiny syringe into a tiny hole in a tiny vial filled with a special kind of sterilized water, sucking it up, then pushing it into *another* equally tiny vial with an equally tiny hole. Then, I was supposed to go get a new needle that was even *smaller*, suck up the mixture in the second vial, and muster up the courage to jab it somewhere into my subcutaneous fat. Between each step, I was supposed to use alcohol wipes to sterilize everything.

Stay positive, Brenda, I would remind myself through gritted teeth. This drug was helpful in reducing the frequency of my relapses. But every time I dealt with all those tiny vials and needles and alcohol wipes, I would wonder, *Didn't the makers of this drug ever* talk *to an MS patient?* Because if they had—even once—they would have known that most MS patients have issues with vision, which means they can't see the tiny holes. Most of us have dexterity issues, which makes all the little pieces incredibly hard to manage. And the included information on *how* to administer the drug was not user friendly. There also wasn't anything in there with information about the disease or other ways I could help myself manage it.

This medication was the first of its kind in the treatment of MS, but the challenges it posed were still overwhelming. My disease had no cure, which meant I faced the prospect of dealing with these every-other-day injections for the foreseeable future—if I was lucky. That was a depressing thought.

On top of all that, I had amassed tens of thousands of dollars in medical debt. My dad had paid for everything initially so that Stephanie and I wouldn't be homeless. Homelessness was a real possibility for MS patients, I had learned. I was meeting people with chronic illnesses that were living on the street. At the time, insurance companies could refuse to cover you and even deny you drugs if you had a preexisting medical condition. If I hadn't been fortunate enough to have a family member in a position to cover my bills, that would have easily been me.

But there was still a pile of debt for me to deal with. *What the hell am I going to do with tens of thousands of dollars' worth of medical bills that I can't pay back?* I thought. I had to come up with some Hail Mary plan.

One evening, when dealing with the tiny little vials and the tiny little needles—a lightbulb went off. I got inspired.

Over the next few days, I tried calling Berlex, the company that made my medication. No one ever picked up the phone. Finally, I called up my dad. "Dad, I need you to drive me over to the pharmaceutical company that makes my drug. I need to tell them why a lot of their stuff isn't helpful for patients and needs improvement. Maybe this could be my job?"

"You're just going to walk in there and make them talk to you?" He chuckled. "Let's go!"

It took us about ninety minutes to get from our home to Richmond, California. I can still remember sitting in traffic—trying to focus on the freeway sounds instead of my anxiety and nervousness. I clutched my cane with sweaty hands. Near the end of the drive, we drove across the San Francisco Bay. In the distance, I could see the Golden Gate bridge. I remembered Dr. Asshole's question to my dad: "If we told your daughter to jump off the Golden Gate bridge, would she?" I stared at that bridge out the left-hand side of the car and thought, *I'm not going to jump off that bridge, you bastard. I was never going to jump off that bridge. There's nothing fucking wrong with me. I have MS.*

The thought reminded me of how far I'd come in the last two and a half years. I gripped my cane and felt some new courage.

When we arrived, I walked up to the door and went up to the reception desk. My dad hung back. I said to the woman behind the desk, "Hello, I am Brenda Snow. I have multiple sclerosis and I take your drug." I took the package out of my purse and stuck it there on the reception counter. "I want to talk to somebody who works on this, because I think there are a lot of things you could be doing differently for patients."

The woman looked at me, taken aback. She said, "Um … Do you want to take a seat?"

"Sure," I said, "But I'd like to know if I can talk to somebody today."

She nodded and touched various papers on the desk as though she was hoping some piece of information there would give her a hint about how to respond. "Why don't you take a seat," she repeated. "I'll be right with you."

We must have sat there for around twenty minutes while the receptionist made hurried calls. She was scrambling. I knew she didn't know what to do with me. If I hadn't been as determined—and as desperate—as I'd been, it would have been the easiest thing to simply tell her, "Here's my name and number. Please have somebody call me when you get the chance." But I was not going to take no for an answer. I *couldn't*.

I wanted to see somebody that day. I wanted to connect with other people like me, with MS. I believed I had *value* I could add to what they were doing. And I was going to give 200 percent of my effort to staying put in that lobby, regardless of how awkward I was making us all feel. Until I had the chance to say my piece and explain why I was there to the right decision maker, I wasn't going anywhere.

Until I had the chance to say my piece and explain why I was there to the right decision maker, I wasn't going anywhere.

Finally, I got my chance. A woman walked out into the lobby from behind the glass. She smiled. "Hi, my name is Michelle," she said warmly. "I work on the Betaseron team. It's incredible to meet you! We've never met a patient before."

I smiled back at her, feeling reassured by her kindness. "I thought that might be the case," I said wryly.

She sat down beside us, right there in the lobby. Over the next half hour, she showed incredible empathy and listening skills while I verbally vomited all over her.

"I think you need a patient focus group," I said. "This packaging doesn't work. These vials and the syringes are very hard to handle for the typical MS patient. Plus, the holes are hard to see with optic neuritis. And *blah blah blah.*" She just listened.

Finally, after I had said everything I wanted to say, Michelle nodded. "Right. I think you've shared some great things here. Let me get your contact information and regroup with my team."

We left. I tried to keep a lid on my excitement. I said to my dad, "Who knows? They'll probably never call." But a bigger part of me thought she would. If it had been anyone else, it probably wouldn't have gone anywhere. But this woman seemed to have all the right stuff. It was obvious Michelle cared deeply about the work she was doing. That was a special time to be in biotech because that drug was the first solution ever for people with relapsing MS. Michelle and her team believed they were taking part in a historic moment.

Deep down, I hoped maybe I was about to take part in one, too.

IT'S TOUGH TO BE AGGRESSIVE WHEN YOU FEEL SICK

That was a good day. It's a good day when you feel strong enough to do something ballsy and aggressive.

Many days are not like that. In this Optimize Your Care phase—where I'm recommending you *pursue,* and *seek,* and be *aggressive,* and *self-advocate*, we need to acknowledge the obvious: all of those action verbs are energy dependent. Some days, you might have it. Some days, you just don't. I'm remembering just how wiped out I was after trying to walk to the mailbox and back during a flare-up. On that day, no way could I storm the castle at a major pharmaceutical maker. On that day, the best I could do to self-advocate was to gently correct my neighbor's assumptions.

But—that was something.

To whatever extent you're able, you need to advocate for yourself right out of the gate—right from the beginning. This is *your* sick story, and *you* should be the one steering the car. But we're also not going to kid ourselves and pretend that our symptoms, side effects, and attacks aren't real. For every patient that reads this book, hear this big, fat, loud validation: in the midst of acute flare-ups or symptoms, aggressive self-advocacy feels fucking impossible. It just does.

To whatever extent you're able, advocate for yourself right out of the gate. This is *your* sick story, and *you* should be the one steering the car.

That's when it's great to have a care partner who can work in tandem with you on your hard days. All the communication we discussed in the previous chapter can help you set up your care partner as a surrogate advocate.

In fact, let's interrupt our regularly scheduled program to bring this message to our care partners.

MESSAGE TO CARE PARTNERS: OPTIMIZE YOUR CARE

There will be many days when a patient doesn't have it in them to be a ballbuster. They won't have the energy to get on the phone and demand what they want. So, guess what?

On those days, *you* get to be the aggressive one.

Remember: both you and your loved one may need to develop this skill of strong self-advocacy. That's not a bad thing. Those new skills are some of the gifts you can expect out of this Journey. Both patients and care partners need to make it known to all the healthcare workers that the care partner is allowed to speak on the patient's behalf. Whether you're working with home help, ancillary healthcare professionals, or your loved one's physician team, communicate that at the beginning. I recommend patients and care partners establish that trusted partnership as early as possible, because the patient's disease and its required medications may cause unpredictable effects. There were times for me when, cognitively, I couldn't understand what the healthcare professionals were even saying. My cognition and memory had been so compromised that they might as well have been speaking Martian. I needed either Melinda or my dad to listen, take notes, and explain it to me later.

Prepare to serve in that role, as needed. *You* may need to be the aggressive one, the primary communicator, or the chief listener and learner. Take notes as needed, or do voice recordings on your phone so that you can relisten to key information from the healthcare team later. Delegate some of these other learning responsibilities to other willing friends or family members, such as researching clinical trials or advocacy organizations.

You're an invaluable support in this information seeking phase, especially when your loved one can't rally to do the hard learning for themselves.

Seek, and Ye Shall Find

In the game of Hide and Seek, the seeker keeps looking until they find the kid they're looking for. You need to have the same attitude with this illness. Keep seeking! *Keep at it*, until you get what you need.

That goes for appointments. If the specialists want to put you off for months, you need to *call in daily* to ask if there have been any cancellations, so that you can get into an appointment sooner. You may need to be a squeaky wheel to get the care you need from an overwhelmed system.

That goes for meds, too. You may need to fight to get yourself on the newest medication. You may need to push to get accepted into a clinical trial. Unfortunately, no one is going to hand you your ideal healthcare treatment on a silver platter. You have to *go after it*.

Where else do you need a fighting spirit? You are entitled to *ask questions* and receive answers from your healthcare team. There is a Patient's Bill of Rights, and asking questions is one of those rights. For some reason, patients and caregivers are often hesitant to ask questions. They're intimidated by the doctors or scared about the disease, so they just accept whatever the doctor tells them is the right course of action. They don't push back. They don't ask follow-up questions.

You are entitled to *ask questions* and receive answers from your healthcare team. There is a Patient's Bill of Rights, and asking questions is one of those rights.

Patients tell me all the time, "I don't want to bother the doctor." *But you should.* You have that right as a patient! Where would I be if I had passively accepted the Asshole Doctor's conclusion that

I was crazy and my daughter should be removed from my care? I don't want to know. Healthcare professionals are fallible people. Second opinions are often warranted. At the very least, you should ask questions until you fully understand and support the recommendations from your health team. And listen to your gut. If it doesn't look right or smell right, it usually isn't right. I know an MS patient who had been dealing with her disease for a while when she suddenly had all kinds of new symptoms. She was rapidly progressing downhill. Her doctors ordered an MRI to check for new lesions on her myelin, but when the results came in, they told her everything looked good. "No new lesions. You're fine," they told her. "You don't need any change in your medication."

A month later, she was still struggling. The family sensed that something wasn't right, and they called up the doctor to ask why she would be experiencing such debilitation if there were no new lesions. The doctors brought up her MRI again.

"Oops—" they said. "We're so sorry. We were looking at the wrong patient chart."

Oops. Oops! Like I said, healthcare professionals are human and fallible.

When they pulled up the correct MRI, they realized this patient *did* have new lesions and required a revised medication plan. One valuable month had expired. But what might have happened if two years had passed and the patient had never addressed these issues? How might she have declined physically if she had decided she "didn't want to bother the doctor"?

You have good reasons to "bother the doctor." Some older generations grew up with the notion that the physician was not to be questioned. But consider where the healthcare system is in the mid-2020s—it's changed a lot over the past sixty years. There's enormous pressure on physicians and hospitals to be profitable, and as a result, appointments are shorter than they used to be, and many systems are understaffed. That's especially true post-pandemic, and these issues unfortunately affect quality of care. I wish this wasn't the case, but it's simply reality. I believe that all of these people are doing the best they can, but they're human. All of us can make mistakes, especially if we're tired and overworked. No one wants to give you suboptimal care—but they're working within a system under pressure.

How do you advocate for yourself in that system? Embrace being a squeaky wheel. Demand the level of care you need. Telehealth is fine if you have a sinus infection, but telehealth won't cut it if you're a cancer patient. Call in until you get an in-person appointment. You don't have to be an asshole about it, but you'll probably need to be persistent. There used to be people appointed as patient advocates within the healthcare system, but these days, that's you.

Advocate for yourself. Be strong for yourself. If you don't show up for you, no one else is going to show up for you.

Advocate for yourself. Be strong for yourself. If you don't show up for you, no one else is going to show up for you. Remember: *you* know your body better than anyone else. Lean into that knowledge and confident headspace; if it doesn't feel right, you are absolutely entitled to push for a better explanation. Be honest with your copilot when things don't feel okay, or if you need them to take the lead on a day when you're not 100 percent. Keep in mind: even *that* requires you to self-advocate and admit, "I need some help here." It is your job to communicate that. And you can! You're a badass sickie.

Here's the moral of the story: you as a patient need to advocate for yourself, with whatever energy you can muster. Listen to your gut and raise your voice. It's your right.

PATIENT PERSPECTIVE: MARNINA M., HIV

The mere sight of a white lab coat and the scent of rubber gloves used to send shivers down my spine. Medical settings were a realm I felt uncomfortable exploring, marked by an aura of anxiety and uncertainty. However, life has a way of surprising us. As a person living with a chronic manageable illness, I began my journey toward well-being; I discovered a different side of healthcare—one focused on prevention and holistic measures rather than just treating ailments. Upon realizing that my well-being required more than just routine doctor visits, I embarked on the transformative journey of health optimization.

As a Black woman living with HIV in the American South, navigating healthcare comes with a history of justified mistrust within the communities I occupy. The echoes of systemic disparities and historical injustices create understandable skepticism. However, amidst this uncertainty, a transformative shift occurred; it led me toward being an active participant in my healthcare when I realized that my healthcare plan must start and end with me.

In my role as an HIV Activist, I have the privilege of sharing this transformative perspective with so many of my peers. This outlook empowers me to take control of my health and reclaim agency over my body. I turned a legacy of mistrust into a journey of empowerment. It's a testament to resilience and a step toward dismantling barriers that have long hindered equitable healthcare access.

In embracing the concept of health optimization, I have a new-found sense of control over my well-being, turning a once dreaded subject into a journey of self-discovery and empowerment. I only get one body during this lifetime. I'm determined to treat it with care.

CONNECT WITH THE RIGHT PEOPLE

Now, let's talk about the kind of information you need to seek out. By far the biggest category won't be "what" but "who." Connecting with the right people will not only connect you with the right information (since the best people will also have the best information), but it will also help optimize your healthcare plan in every respect.

There's a lot of people you're going to want to seek out. Are you ready? Take a deep breath. Let's dive in.

Healthcare Professionals

Your first priority in the Optimize Your Care phase is to ensure you're meeting with the right healthcare team. Or teams. "Healthcare professionals" is a wide bucket and includes some or all of the following:

- **Your primary specialist:** Whatever disease you have, there will be one main doctor who leads the coordination of your care. If you're a cancer patient, that will be your oncologist. If you have MS, like me, that would be your neurologist. Whoever this person is, you want them to be a shining star in their field.

- **Your primary care physician (PCP):** This person will remain a key fixture on your team, even though most of your disease-specific treatments will be handled by specialists. But if you live somewhere like rural Iowa, you may be hundreds of miles away from an institution that treats the unique disease you have. All of your day-to-day disease management will be with your PCP, working in tandem with your specialist(s). Many people, once launched into the Patient's Journey, assume they'll never need their PCP again, but you will get other symptoms or illnesses as a patient, and you need to stay on top of them. When you contract a cold and you're immunocompromised: you start with your PCP. When you cut your hand while slicing into an avocado and you know you have a heightened risk of infection: you start with your PCP. Ideally, your PCP will be someone who makes themselves available to you, takes your symptoms seriously, and will pursue new knowledge as needed.

- **Nurses:** Your team will include an entire sphere of them. Your physician will have a team of nurses; there will be a different set of nurses that administer your infusions or your chemotherapy; there are specialized nurses called health educators who might provide tailored instruction in a certain area, like if you are preparing to get an organ transplant or preparing to begin a complex medical treatment; and there are also nursing support staff. You won't have the opportunity to choose your nurses, but it's still your obligation to speak up for yourself if you have feedback or concerns about their method of care.

- **Ancillary specialists:** This part of the "bucket" includes all the other people who are key participants in your care but perhaps not right at the center of your treatment. We're talking physical therapists, cognitive therapists, occupational therapists, mental health support, and so on. Ideally, you want ancillary specialists who are good at their job, kind, and available.
- **Another specialist:** Many diseases require additional specialists. For instance, although my primary specialist was a neurologist, I also had significant bladder issues for a long time and needed to see a urologist as well. If you're a bone cancer patient, you might need an orthopedic surgeon on your team, or a radiation specialist, in addition to your main oncologist. Whoever these additional specialists are, you want to find people who will stay in communication with your primary specialist and PCP to ensure good coordination of care. (This is an area where you can advocate for yourself: request their regular communication.)

It's a lot. But take another deep breath—we're not done yet.

Therapeutics

Another major area where you'll need to school yourself is the category of therapeutics and medications. When I was diagnosed in 1993, there wasn't a single FDA-approved drug for relapsing forms of MS. When one finally came on the market, my choice was simple: I could choose to take it or not. In 2023, there are now over *twenty-two* approved therapies. A new MS patient has a much more complex set of choices to make about what therapy they choose for themselves, and physicians don't always have a clear recommendation about which one will be the best.

In many ways, this is a great problem to have; for many illnesses, patients don't have the option to choose. However, in the last few decades, there's been enormous, accelerated progress in the biotech field and an increasing number of diagnoses now have multiple options for treatment. Many diseases that were thought to be untreatable are now treatable; some "incurable" diseases now have a cure. The improvement in breast cancer mortality statistics alone is jaw-dropping. So, while the advancement of science has provided patients with many great choices, those choices still pose a challenge for the patient. How to choose?

I tend to see two things happen for patients when choosing a medication.

Situation A: The doctors give you almost no choice. Instead, they do all the choosing for you. When it comes to oncology for instance, the cocktails of drugs that need to work together for specific cancers tend to be highly sophisticated. Really, the only people qualified to issue recommendations about the combination of immunotherapies, chemotherapeutic agents, and any other therapies that may be required are the specialists on your team. This is especially true if you're getting into gene therapy—which requires the expertise of a trained physician.

Sometimes—ideally—your team of doctors will take your case to a review board within their health system, present your case, and voice the recommendations they're thinking about. Then, their colleagues have a chance to weigh in and your doctors get the benefit of peer review. That's the "Mercedes-Benz" of therapeutic recommendations, and it occurs most in cases where a life is on the line.

Situation B: The doctors give you almost no guidance. On the other hand, there are many other non-life-threatening diseases that, while still serious, aren't likely to kill you: diseases like psoriasis, rheumatoid arthritis, multiple sclerosis, epilepsy, psoriatic arthritis, different thyroid conditions, and so on. In the last few decades, most of these diseases have now acquired a large number of highly advanced therapeutics for treatment. And when it's time for you to choose what particular therapeutic you want prescribed, many doctors don't want to pick it for you. They'll say, "Here are the choices. Pick which one you want and let me know." I don't know why doctors hold back on recommending medications—and if I had a nickel for every time someone asked me why their doctor wouldn't help them pick a therapy, I'd have a good-sized piggy bank. But I have some theories.

First, your doctor may not be incredibly familiar with your disease. It's not like you're walking in with the flu, and they're treating several hundred people in the same week with the same flu. Your doctor—even a specialist—may have only seen a few other people with your disease. They may not have gathered enough experience to feel confident about which therapies work best.

Another theory why a physician might hold off on a recommendation is because all of the therapies look equally effective. Each medication might do about the same thing. And your physician might know that you, as the patient, are more likely to *stay consistent* with your treatment if you're allowed to be the captain of the ship. If a patient comes in and says, "I hate needles. I can't take medication with a needle, no way," then it makes sense for that patient to choose a comparable medication that comes in pill form. And that patient is likely to be more compliant and get their disease managed by taking pills, rather than dealing with shots or an infused product. It could also be that your doctor just wants to cover their ass. Making a choice always entails the risk of getting it wrong initially, regardless of risk profiles and the level of research you've put into it. Nobody wants to be the one who got it wrong. Regardless of why you may not get a straightforward recommendation, it can be overwhelming for a patient when there's nobody narrowing down the choices for them. I've seen many patients get handed a bunch of pamphlets, brochures, and/or websites at a time in their disease when they're tired, stressed, and nervous. And that's a lot of shit to try to read and digest when you don't feel well.

This is a great time to advocate for yourself *if* you have the energy, or delegate research to a friend. Here are some of the key terms you'll want to consider when selecting a medication:

- **Efficacy:** First and foremost, you want a drug that *works* for you. Look at clinical trials for these numbers. Did this medication show a 30 percent reduction in new symptoms, or a 70 percent reduction in new symptoms? If you have the option to choose a more effective treatment over one that's had less success, that might be an obvious indicator for you.

- **Safety:** Safety encompasses three things: side effects, contraindications, and drug interactions. *Side effects:* Just about every medication will come with some side effects—it's the price you pay for the drug's efficacy. Pay attention to the side effects profile and consider which ones you can and can't live with. *Contraindications:* This big, fat word mainly refers to a negative impact you might experience from the drug due to allergies or another underlying conditions. For instance, I had anaphylactic shock from a medication that we didn't know was contraindicated for me. *Drug interactions:* Most patients with a chronic condition are taking multiple medications, so you need to make sure they play nice together. If the drugs interplay in a negative way, they could cancel out each other's efficacy and/or increase unpleasant side effects.

- **Convenience and dosage form:** How will you take the medication? Is it a pill? A shot? Is it infused? And what frequency is required? Is this a medication you have to take once a year, every six months, or once every day? Can you take it at home, or do you have to add visits to the clinic to your appointment schedule? Sometimes, you're stuck with an injectable, but often you may have more options. Consider your preferences for route of administration, but *second to efficacy*—efficacy is more important. If you're facing something like cancer, you may not get much of a choice about how you take your drug. But if you're dealing with a chronic condition, you'll be most successful with a medication you can take consistently and conveniently. Be honest with yourself about whether or not you can handle a particular drug's dosage form.

- **Insurance coverage and cost:** Insurance coverage can sometimes determine which treatment you will receive. Occasionally there is wiggle room, but wiggling will always require phone calls and sometimes letters or outside help. In many cases, insurers will demand that you first try a more economical drug before they approve you for the drug you really need or want. "Step therapy" is the euphemistic name for this practice. It's one of those unfortunate situations where a third party gets to make rules that aren't designed to empower you. Remember what you learned in the Endurance chapter and keep fighting for what you need. Also, know that the sooner you start and the quicker you move through the process, the sooner you'll get to your destination.

- **Patient reviews and physician recommendations:** If you pay attention to five-star reviews for your Friday night restaurant, why wouldn't you look into reviews for a medication you're injecting into your body? Seek out information about other patients' experiences and reactions to the drug you're considering. Work collaboratively with your doctor in choosing a treatment, but if you have any concerns, don't be afraid to push back and pursue a second opinion about an alternate medication.

When you as a patient can start to make sense of these different categorical features and begin to identify what you're willing to do or not do, you'll find increased clarity amidst all the clutter.

And once you do, you'll feel an increased sense of empowerment. I've heard patients say, "Because there are so many drugs out there and I'm really doing pretty well at this point, compared to most people with the disease, I'm going to start taking the drug that showed thirty-five percent efficacy in the clinical trial because it had the mildest side effects. I'll save the bigger gun, the medication with seventy percent efficacy, for further down the road if I need to give my disease a punch in the face." Remarks like that typically indicate the patient has done a lot of research into the specifics of their therapeutic options and has made a choice that they feel confident about.

Learning the specifics of your therapeutic options will help you feel empowered.

Keep in mind that any therapeutic decisions should be made with your healthcare professionals. Ideally, you'll get some guidance from your physicians about what medications they've seen be most successful, but it's also valuable for you to assert some agency in the process as well.

Other Professionals

What else do you need to know? *Who* else do you need to know? Let's add a few more bullet points to the list of whos and whats you'll want to learn about:

- **Mental health support:** For obvious reasons.
- **The person who knows about social security and disability (SSDI):** Dealing with all this fine print is a

fucking nightmare, but it's critical information to piece together if you're not working. Try seeking out help from a social worker affiliated with the nonprofit organization associated with your illness. For me, that was the National MS Society. They directed me to a lawyer who provided pro bono help to MS patients; with his help, I was able to apply for these benefits. (Obviously, once I went back to work, I no longer took the benefits.) These social workers function as your air traffic control: they won't do the legwork for you, but they can direct you to people in their network who *can* provide help. That would be a good first stop to gather initial information. Additionally, sometimes when you apply for SSDI, you'll be assigned a caseworker. If you're lucky, you'll get someone helpful who can answer questions or point you toward resources. Alternately, you may need to recruit someone from your own network who can help wade through all of this with you. Most people will benefit hugely from having an "expert" in this area on your team. Some people will have the skills to navigate the fine print of social security and disability on their own, but *I* was not one of those people.

- **The person who knows about insurance:** Another fucking nightmare. You have insurance, your spouse has insurance, your parents have you on their insurance; never mind, you have no insurance. Whatever your insurance situation—it needs to be figured out. If you're covered by two forms of insurance, you might be able to benefit from two kinds of coverage. If you have *no* insurance, you need to work with a team that will help you figure out how to find and get insurance. In some cases, you might have to rely on patient support programs and services to get free coverage of medications or free services.

- **Legal help:** Because of all the red tape mentioned above, sometimes the help you need and have a legal right to *doesn't* arrive, and then you need to call in the lawyers. Who has the money at this point to hire attorneys? Not everybody can go this route, but for some people, it's another necessary person to seek out. Remember that legal help may be available through nonprofit organizations that advocate for patients exactly like you.

On top of all this, you need a new filing system at home, just to keep all the paperwork organized. It's a *lot* to manage.

Deep breath. I know it can seem overwhelming.

So, here's my advice: look at this in digestible courses. There's an order of operations: first *who*, then *what*, and finally *how*. Get your healthcare team in place, because then you've got trusted professionals helping you make some of these other decisions. With their guidance, get your *what*: medications, therapies, and all the rest. Finally, you're going to tackle the *how,* in dealing with insurance, paperwork, social security, etc.

And if you still feel overwhelmed to the point that you'd like to throw this book at the wall—maybe go back to Chapter 4 and read about the power of positivity. Remember that it gets better! It gets easier. You *will* get through it.

But you're going to have to have the patience of Job.

**It gets better! It gets easier. You *will* get through it.
But you're going to have to have the patience of Job.**

Also, you're going to need to raise your hand and alert your community to your need for help. (I have no problem repeating this advice. I suspect you need it repeated.) Lean into your family and friends for help navigating these different areas. Be 100 percent transparent with them that you're overwhelmed and need help making phone calls, reading through the stuff, choosing the medication, and so on.

There are also people out there who do this for a living. They can help, too.

Advocacy and Civic Organizations

One valuable way to expend your limited energy and time is by seeking out advocacy organizations that can help you do everything I just talked about. For example, there are wonderful advocacy groups such as patientadvocate.org, which offers case management support (insurance denials, healthcare access issues, medical debt challenges), co-pay relief programs, small financial aid grants, and access to a national financial resource directory. These sorts of advocacy organizations can help you wade through social security, disability benefits, insurance coverage, supplemental insurance, co-pays on drugs—*and all the things.*

Civic organizations are another great source to look into for help—for instance, your local Kiwanis Club, Rotary Club, Lion's

Club, or even the YMCA. Many of these groups have volunteers who can provide assistance with some of the logistical headaches—filling out forms, arranging for medicine to be delivered, providing short term transportation, renewing assistance programs, and so on. Try calling the club's president or officers to find out if that's a volunteer service they offer.

One valuable way to expend your limited energy and time is by seeking out advocacy organizations that can help you navigate fine print and/or the complexities of healthcare.

Also, I recommend you seek out whatever society is related to your disease. For instance, I was able to access pro bono legal advice through the National Multiple Sclerosis Society. Many of these disease-specific societies have similar services, along with people on their staff who donate their time to help patients navigate all the information they need to know.

Yes—it's one more thing to seek out. But these advocacy and civic organizations can end up saving you time and energy (and often, money, too) in the long run. On the days when you feel overwhelmed, take comfort in the fact that help is available. Once you feel up to making yet another phone call—try one of these organizations.

Clinical Trials

Last one: many patients also find it worth their while to seek out clinical trials to participate in. The scientific world is generating new treatments all the time and there may be a new therapy for your disease that's currently under research. But it's important to understand that in most clinical trials, the drug is tested against placebo, so there's a chance you're not actually receiving *any* real medication while data is collected. Make sure you know what you can and cannot expect and that you can handle the uncertainty.

This will require a fair amount of research on your part, but for some patients, *that's* where they believe they'll get the greatest return on their investment of time and energy. Two useful websites if you want to explore this option further:

- **ClincialTrials.gov:** This site will let you enter a variety of criteria to look for clinical trials that might relate to your specific needs, such as the name of your disease and/or a medication you want to read about. You can also narrow your search to look up studies currently recruiting patients if you think you'd like to participate in a clinical trial. Alternatively, you can use this database as a quick go-to spot to learn more about your disease, potential medications, and/or available therapies.

- **Patientworthy.com:** This site was created by Snow Companies for patients with rare diseases to connect with one another and learn more about their particular diagnosis. You'll find a search bar on the home landing page where you can type in your disease. The search results will provide you with a mixture of patient stories and research, enabling you to both connect with other patients and learn cutting-edge information about your disease.

DEFINE AND REFINE THE PLAN

Now that you've sought out the people you need on your team and have learned key information about your disease and therapeutics, it's time for you to take the lead on forming your plan. Once again, you're going to need to put on your big kid pants and advocate for yourself in this area. Be empowered! You've worked hard to seek out good information. The more you learn about each aspect of your patient plan, the more knowledge you can apply in terms of what will be best for *you*.

Once you have your plan, I want you to practice marching into your doctor's office, holding it up, and saying, "I need this plan to work because I want my life to be good. So, get out of my fucking way."

Seriously, practice this at home. Look in the mirror and holler out, "Get out of my fucking way!" You'll feel terrific. The point being: put yourself in the driver's seat. Make your plan, and once you've got it sorted, don't let others mess it all up again. Be confident in your decisions! You don't have control over much in your life right now, but you *do* have control over your treatment and healthcare team. As you assert your agency, enjoy mustering this modicum of control. It will help you feel better!

Here are the areas where *you* get to take charge and be the primary decision maker:

Assess Your Team

- Is your doctor the right doctor? Are their nursing staff helpful? Do you have a productive relationship with this team? Are they giving you the time that you need?

Are they answering your questions? Are they validating you? Are they referencing the most cutting-edge information?

Assess Your Therapeutics

- Do you feel confident about the medication you've chosen?
- Do you know how to administer the medication? (E.g., you've been trained if it's an injectable or infused product.) Have you been educated on the possible side effects and how you can best mitigate them? Do you feel supported by healthcare professionals and know who to ask questions about your medication, when they arise?
- Do you know the schedule and rhythm of your treatment(s)? For instance, how many down days should you expect after a chemo treatment? Is that same information being provided to your care partner(s) and support team? Do they know what to do when you're yakking your guts out four days in a row?

Assess Your Rehabilitation Therapies

- When do you need rehabilitation therapies? Do you need a speech therapist, a cognitive therapist, a physical or occupational or mental health therapist? Or maybe a pelvic floor physical therapist (raising my hand) or an audio therapist? The list could go on and on.

- What's the schedule of your therapy appointments? How many times are you going per week? Does this schedule work with the rhythm of your medical treatments?
- Do you feel happy with your therapy team(s)? Are they listening to you? Do they make you feel supported and encouraged? Do you feel optimistic that they can help you progress?

Assess the Financial Stuff

- Is your medical insurance covering your bills? Are the bills getting paid? Are your *other* bills getting paid?
- Do you need to lean into other forms of support to help pay for some of your medical bills?

Assess the Life Logistics Stuff

- What areas of your life are showing strain? Where do you need to call in extra support?
- Would it be helpful to have meals provided? Who can you call to drive your kids around if/when you're feeling especially ill? Who's going to the grocery store? Who's feeding your family? Who's doing the chores?
- What's your plan for tracking, storing, and organizing your medications?
- What's your plan for going on vacation?
- Will you reenter the workforce? When and how? What do you need to communicate to your employers? Who

at your workplace will you tell about your disease? If you intend to not communicate about your illness, what are the ramifications of that?

By making choices around each of these aspects of your plan, you put yourself in the driver's seat. That's powerful! And—calling back to the message of Chapter 4—this is why it's so critical to operate with positivity: *so that you can make choices that reflect hope for a better future.* Make choices that will take you toward wellness. Make choices that will help you chase the light at the end of the tunnel.

Make choices that reflect hope for a better future.

Make those hope-filled choices, *even if your diagnosis is terminal.* In fact, there's one more element of the plan that you'd do well to think about:

Assess Your End-of-Life Options

- Are your personal affairs in order? If not, who do you need to seek out to help you organize your estate? Is your will or trust up to date?
- Do you need a medical advance directive? Do you want a DNR (do not resuscitate) order? Do you have a person designated as your power of attorney?
- Does your family know your wishes about what kind of memorial service you want?

Once again—hold off before throwing this book against the wall. Many people consider it disturbing to consider their own death, but this is also an area where patients might recognize it as more *necessary* than they ever have before. And I will challenge you to think of these end-of-life considerations as an opportunity to *love* your family and reflect *joyfully* on your life.

Here's what I mean. My mom is currently eighty years old (though, according to her, she's seventy). I call her the Queen of Fun, because from my earliest memories, she's been the life of the party. She makes everything exciting. Maybe that's why things like death are taboo for her since death isn't exactly the most fun or exciting topic. She has never, ever wanted to discuss end-of-life stuff. Finally, I said to her, "Mom, I know this is super depressing, but we need to know what you want. We want to honor you well!"

Even though Mom didn't want to talk about it, she finally agreed to write everything down. She gave my sister and me a manila folder with all of her details written down on pages inside.

My sister read it first. She drew a "sad face" emoji on it. When she gave it to me, she said, "This is a depressing day."

I said, "Well, yeah. Nobody wants to think about these things." But when I read through the document, I had a completely different take. My mom—the Queen of Fun—had injected fun into every bit of her end-of-life planning. She'd written things like, "When I'm dead, I want a ballroom dancing party. I only want music played by Elvis. Serve cheeseburgers and make it like a 1950s soda fountain." I ended up laughing out loud at some of her requests. She was going to keep the party going even after her death, and I just love her for it.

That's an attitude you can choose! If you're reading this book and thinking, "Wow, this is a depressing subject"—just think about the *control* you could exert in this process! As someone who loves control, I get excited thinking about *my* end-of-life plan. I'm like, "Wow, I get the opportunity to control things from the grave!" Nothing excites me more than having the last word. Your end-of-life plan is the biggest and best opportunity to be a control freak to the bitter end and beyond.

My point is that, with every aspect of your plan, you will determine how you frame it. You can either see this process as overwhelming and impossible, or you can view it as an opportunity to take the reins and become a more empowered patient. You can view your end-of-life planning as a miserable, morbid exercise, or you can delight in crafting a memorable experience that will sing out your legacy and enable others to celebrate you, whenever your time finally comes.

When seeking out information that will help you form your healthcare plan, you can either see this process as overwhelming and impossible, or you can view it as an opportunity to take the reins and become a more empowered patient.

It's also important to consider the consequences of *failing* to plan. I don't say this to bum you out, but to inform you: *not* planning in any of these areas can have serious ramifications. In some states, if you die and have no will, that can put your estate and your family in real jeopardy. I'm sure you care deeply about your family and seek to protect them in every way you can. You should have that same attitude toward them in matters related to your death. Wouldn't you want them to continue to be protected after you're gone? If so, you need to be proactive in getting your affairs together. It's as simple as that for me.

So, once you have a plan pulled together and defined, *revisit it*. Refine it. Hone it. If your doctor proves to be an asshole or an imbecile, refine that part of the plan! I can't tell you how many doctors I've fired: "Sorry, you didn't give me the time of day. You're out of here. I'm going to find someone else." Get a new doctor in place and tweak your plan.

If you graduate beyond a certain therapy because you can do all the things now, refine the plan. Take that appointment off your calendar.

If you're not doing well on a certain medication, refine the plan. Set yourself up to incorporate a new medication.

If your son divorces your daughter-in-law and you want to make changes in your will, refine the plan. Call up an estate lawyer and make sure all the names in your will or trust are current.

Remember: you are a badass sickie. You *can* be aggressive. You are your own best advocate. And YOU get to choose the plan that will take you toward greater health, hope, and wholeness.

You have strength in you that you haven't even discovered yet.

Don't think you can do it? I didn't either. But you've got strength in you that you haven't even discovered yet. And when you put yourself out there as your own advocate, you might just find it.

STANDING STORYTELLER

I wasn't sure I would ever hear from the Betaseron people again. But I *did*.

A few days after I stormed the castle at Berlex, I got a call from Michelle. "Brenda, we'd love for you to come in and meet with the entire Berlex team," she said.

"The Betaseron team?" I asked.

She corrected me. "The Berlex team. The entire company. Would you be able to share more about what you told me? The way the drug has helped you and some of your thoughts on how to make it better?" Elated, I agreed. We set up a date.

Then, I hung up the phone. I realized what I had just committed myself to.

Ooooh shit, I thought. *Shitshitshittyshit.* The prospect of giving a speech to the entire Berlex company scared me to death.

As the day got closer and I worked on my story, my intrinsic motivation to "wow" them went through the roof. I tend to be a procrastinator normally, but I wanted to do this *well*. I wanted to move everyone in that room to an emotional place where they would never forget me. I knew—if I could do that—it might make all those scientists go back to their labs and strive to do even better at their work. It could bring more meaning and purpose to their jobs. At the time, I thought they might even be able to come up with a cure. *If I do my job well enough and I move these people to the place I want them to get to, maybe I'll see a cure in my lifetime.* That's what I thought. That's what was at stake.

So, I dressed up. I had gained a lot of weight from the steroids and obviously wasn't able to do a lot of exercise at the time, but I wore a black skirt, a nice top, and a fitted, fake Burberry plaid jacket with a zipper that my mom had picked out for me. Mom knew I felt self-conscious about how my body had physically changed since I'd gotten MS, and she's a style icon—I think she knew that zipping me up in that jacket would give me a little extra confidence.

I also prepped my visuals. At that time in the '90s, laptops existed, but I hate computers. However, I *had* done quite a bit of volunteering in Stephanie's classroom at that point and had seen lots of teaching with the overhead projector. So, I got myself some overhead projector sheets. I made ten topic points. I fancy myself a crappy artist, so I had made a mixed media collage to show different phases in my MS journey up to that point. There were pictures of me with my walker and my cane in the hospital; there was a picture of me giving a talk to the MS Society. In the middle of all the pictures, I had an image of the Betaseron box and logo. *This might make them feel good to see*, I thought. *To see a lady that's had success with their drug.*

Last of all, I practiced standing with my cane. At the time, I was not a full-time walker, and my legs were still quite weak. I used an ambulation device—either a walker or a cane—and never stood for long. But it was very important to me that I *start* my presentation standing and *finish* standing. I was still working through what it meant to be a young woman using devices that mostly old people used. The wheelchair, to me, felt associated with the hardest months of my sickness. The walker felt like a means to an end. But the cane felt more like "baller status." I could stand there with a cane and be like, "That's right, this is how I roll."

On the day of the presentation, I walked into a large blue multiuse room. I was relieved to see that the lighting was low—bright lights were tough on my optic neuritis. There were several hundred people who had gathered themselves into different teams— marketing, operations, science. I saw a section of people in lab coats, just like all the physicians I'd seen. The haze of my fear was briefly interrupted when I saw them. I thought, *That's funny. None of them are physicians but they wear the same symbol of authority. Let's hope these people are better at their jobs than some of those doctors were at diagnosing me!* I was so nervous. Even though I had some experience as a speaker and had shared my story about MS with plenty of people by then, I didn't know if I could get a word out. I felt so much fear. The palms of my hands were slippery with sweat. As they prepared to introduce me, I rubbed my hands together for a few seconds, imagined all my nervous energy, then released my hands as though I was throwing all that energy out into the room. I took a deep breath. They said my name and I stood up.

This is your moment, Brenda, I thought. *This is where you could change your life and change other people's lives.* I paused, smiled at the audience, and gave myself one more stern mental warning: *Don't fuck up!*

I talked for about forty-five minutes. I first shared about my initial symptoms, what it was like to try to get a diagnosis, and how horribly I was treated by the medical community. (Shout out to Dr. Asshole!) I talked about what it was like to lie in a hospital bed and wonder if I was ever going to get up. I described what it was like to pee myself in the Macy's dressing room, and what it was like to have my daughter push my wheelchair across the intersection to get to her kindergarten. I shared about what it really looks like to live with a chronic illness.

I shared about what it really looks like to live with a chronic illness.

Then, I juxtaposed all of that with descriptions of some of my restored health, as a result of taking their drug. At the time, a lot of MS patients were still nervous about taking Betaseron. Just like there was some skepticism with the coronavirus vaccine in its early days, people were nervous that the drug didn't have a long history. Everyone wondered what the hell they were injecting. "In my mind," I explained, "It was either Betaseron, or I'm back in a wheelchair in ten years without the option of ever getting up again. There was no other option. That's why I was willing to take the risk. And now it's paying off."

I told the Berlex team that I'd been telling people at MS support groups about my success with their drug. But I also poked fun at all the aspects of the drug that were irritating to me: the tiny holes, the tiny tubes, the tiny needles, and so on. I got some laughs.

It was also important to me to share about everything else I was doing to achieve progress: physical therapy three times a week, occupational therapy twice a week. "Sleep is mega-hugely impor-tant for me," I said, "I get between nine and ten hours of sleep per night. I utilized complementary therapies. *And* I take Betaseron. The drug is part of a multidisciplinary approach with lots of differ-ent modalities that has literally gotten me back on my feet. And I think those are things your patient population would benefit from hearing about. It would benefit your marketing if you did more patient education, because people are desperate to know this stuff."

Halfway through the presentation, I sat down briefly in a chair they'd set beside me. But other than that, I stood.

It was brutal—*brutal*—but I stood almost the entire time.

I felt so much gratitude and hope. I said, "I really hope you are the people who are going to crack the code. I really hope you can make life better for people with chronic illness, and specifically multiple sclerosis."

Michelle hurried up to me afterward, beaming. "Amazing," she whispered. "Resounding success. And now, we're taking you on a tour of the lab."

I loved touring the lab—it made me feel proud and excited about the work they were doing. When we got to the area where the drugs were packaged up, I teased them about my inability to see the vials. When they asked me questions, I would say something like, "I don't know, because I can't pop off the top!" They laughed and the walls came down, but it was clear to all of us that the whole thing needed to get better. I learned later that changing the packaging wasn't a simple manufacturing fix; the packaging was part of how the FDA approved the drug, so a redesign to the drug's packaging and method of administration would require new regulatory reviews.

Still, they started working on it. They knew the packaging sucked and that it wasn't patient friendly.

After the lab tour, Michelle introduced me to her boss, Paul, who was in charge of the brand. I pitched a patient focus group and suggested they put together more patient education materials. "You need to put more information into patients' hands—information that will show patients you care about them as *people*, not just consumers of your drug."

"What kind of information?" Paul asked.

"You know ... 'How to talk to my kid about my diagnosis.' What about intimacy? What about family planning? Educating patients on how to help mitigate their symptoms, beyond just taking the drug. Stuff like that."

Paul looked at Michelle skeptically, then back at me. "That's not really our role," he said.

"Well, no one *else* is putting out that information," I retorted. "And it's something patients need and something they would value, and if *you're* the brand that gets them that information, that makes you guys look pretty good."

I took a deep breath to make one more big ask. I still had medical bills to pay, and I hadn't forgotten my plan to get them to hire me as a consultant. "One last thing," I told them. "I think you should start flying me around the country to speak to groups of people and share my story. And I'm going to tell them the steps I've taken that have helped me and my MS."

Amazingly, that's what they did. That was the official start of my budding career as a consultant. Sometimes I spoke to a group of patients; sometimes I went to a nonprofit; sometimes I spoke with a group of doctors. I felt like I might be making a difference. And the patients I was meeting were making a difference in *my* life. More than ever before, I realized that I wasn't alone.

In sharing my story, I felt like I might be making a difference. And the patients I was meeting were making a difference in *my* life. More than ever before, I realized that I wasn't alone.

Paul and Michelle also agreed to let me put together a patient focus group, like I'd asked. Over the next few months, we assembled patient education materials. Eventually, I was able to put those in the hands of other MS patients, who had been just as desperate for information as I had been.

Storming the Berlex castle paid off. Within a few years, there was a new and improved Betaseron, thanks to the patient focus group they allowed me to start, and all my squeaky-wheeliness. MS patients around the country were getting better information. I slowly, *slowly* began paying down my debt. And my disease no longer felt like a life-ruining burden. It started feeling like it might possibly—just *possibly*—be a vehicle for impact.

SOMETHING NEW AND BEAUTIFUL

I've given you a lot to think about in this chapter. I wanted to spotlight every area where you'll want to seek out information, because I think it's important to know what you don't know.

But if it's caused you to feel overwhelmed or disheartened, I get it. It's a *lot*.

People talk about "work/life balance," which is a bit of a laugh when you get a chronic or terminal diagnosis. Whatever "balance" may have existed on the scales before now goes out the window. The scale with the illness on it just goes down, down, down, because this disease requires so *much* of your time and energy to deal with.

Listen: from the time you get diagnosed and onward—life won't be balanced. But it will be okay. It *will* be okay.

You will find your new normal. You will pull together your plan. You will learn the things you need to learn. And over time, it will all get easier. I promise you, 100 percent, it *does* get easier.

Eventually, you will find yourself doing things in this new sick version of your life that you would have never imagined yourself doing before. Things that matter—things that make a *difference*.

You will do things that wake you up to the fact that, in this strange new reality, you're building something new and beautiful.

STAGE 8 OF THE PATIENT'S JOURNEY: OPTIMIZE YOUR CARE

- *Common emotions: drive to connect, fear of rejection, desire to organize the chaos that entered your life, feeling overwhelmed.*
- *Common pitfalls: resignation, passivity, victim's attitude.*
- *Your best next step: Claim your rightful place in the driver's seat. You're the pilot-in-command, and you're free to engage the copilots of your choice.*

CHAPTER 10

Rebuilding

ARCHITECTING FUN AND PURPOSE BACK INTO YOUR LIFE

"They say I can't dance anymore. Well, they can go to hell."

— My mom

In the Rebuilding stage of the Patient's Journey, you get to take back happy.

Do you want to know the first way to embrace joy and fun? Give yourself *permission* to do it. Having a disease is a heavy, serious thing. But I've seen people go further than they need to and take on an affect that their whole life has to be serious. It doesn't. Sometimes patients need to be reminded that it's okay to feel good.

Hey. It's okay to feel good!

Your life is not over. Your life is *different*, yes, but not over. And the lives of your loved ones are not over. There's still living to be done! It's not going to be easy. You may have realized after Chapter 7 that it's going to be a hell of a lot of hard work. But the last time I checked, most of the things that require hard work are also incredibly rewarding.

Give yourself permission to have fun! It's okay to feel good.

So now, it's time to figure out how to rebuild your life. You're going to learn how to architect joy into daily living. You're going to take risks that align with your new capabilities and sense of mission. And you're going to do everything possible to milk every moment for happiness.

Reinvention may also be a part of this stage as you discover new purpose, passion, or a sense of mission on the other side of your diagnosis. That was true for me. In my own Patient's Journey, I began rebuilding my life by building a company.

DISCOVERING A PLATFORM

I started traveling around the country, sharing my MS story and speaking about my experiences. Very quickly, there were indicators that this was causing ripple effects in the patient community. A nurse friend told me anecdotally, "Sharing your story is making a difference for MS patients. The patient materials are good, but what's really resonating is the power of your story. Patients who heard your talk are joining support groups, asking questions about different medications—they're empowered! They're taking control." This probably doesn't surprise anyone now in the age of social media influencers, but at the time, the storytelling approach was brand new.

I went back to Paul and Michelle. "We need to tell more stories," I told them. "We need to find more people like me."

They believed me—but pharmaceutical companies are risk averse and working with patients was novel. "Let's focus on getting more nurses on board," they said. Two of my nurse friends created a special training curriculum for nurses to get an advanced certification as an "MS Specialist." They traveled around the country training patients on how to take the medication, often going directly to patients' homes. Most MS patients at that time weren't even going to the doctor because they didn't believe help was available. This intervention was a game changer. Essentially, they were providing patients with a lifeline, enabling them to reengage in their care.

As the nurses provided training, I flew out to join them and narrate "a day in the life of a patient." I shared my story, my tips, and my techniques—all the strategies that were helping me. I went back to Berlex and told them what we were seeing. "Anything that goes to a patient should feature a patient," I said. "Not actors or actresses. Not models. People who are living with this disease." As patients responded en masse to these educational efforts, other pharmaceutical marketers began paying attention.

No one was interviewing me at the time, but if they had, I would have said, "No *duh*. This is what patients have been waiting for!"

Several years into doing this work, I'd made a small but mighty name for myself. At the same time, biotech was taking leaps and bounds forward in innovation. During the mid-1990s, there was an explosion of novel therapeutics and medicines, not only for MS but also for other diseases, like psoriatic arthritis, psoriasis, rheumatoid arthritis, and so on. The discovery of how to employ monoclonal antibodies for healing brought a swath of new treatment options to patients. The '90s weren't just about Seinfeld, Friends, and grunge rock—it was also a decade of scientific breakthroughs for novel therapies.

The increase in options was fortunate for me. I had started to develop some side effects to Betaseron—a not uncommon result for patients who have taken a drug for an extended time. A few years ago, there hadn't been a single drug available for people with my illness; now, thankfully, there were multiple options. And I needed a new one.

I thought a drug called Rebif could be beneficial for me. Serono, the drug's maker, had published compelling data showing Rebif's efficacy. Best of all, Rebif was going to be administered via an auto inject tool. Automatic anything in regard to injections sounded good to me.

I got myself into Rebif's autoinjector trial and observed that the medication seemed to work well for my body. And the autoinjector was fantastic. I wasn't grappling with tiny holes or tiny needles anymore—I put a syringe into a machine, and it did all the work for me. I just pushed a button and the shot was done. Wow!

This created some potential professional complications, however. I didn't feel great being the "face of Betaseron" when I wasn't taking their drug anymore.

Would it work to do this for another company? I wondered. I called and asked to speak to the brand director for Rebif. The brand director was a man named Corbin Wood.

Corbin knew of the work Betaseron had been doing to support patients. In fact, he believed in a story-share approach and wanted to expand, amplify, and create greater structure around patient stories. I didn't know any of this at the time. All I knew was that Corbin Wood, Rebif Brand Director, was willing to meet me for lunch at Legal Seafood in Boston.

True to form, I barely let him get a word in edgewise. Corbin is a great listener and a man of few words. He's also got a killer poker face. That made me nervous, which meant I talked even more than usual!

"I've been working inside patient communities and sharing my story and tips is serving a lot of unmet needs." I spoke quickly and animatedly. Corbin silently ate his lunch. "Traditional biotech and life science companies don't put enough focus on patients. And I think that's shortsighted. Patients need to know what to *do* with the medications they've been prescribed. Whether it's a drug for cancer or a drug for MS, the patient should understand why and how to take it, what it does and doesn't do ... "

Corbin continued to stare at me. I talked faster.

" ... Its side effects, its benefits, how you get the drug paid for ... At the end of the day, the *patient* is the one who needs to buy in. Because if they don't understand the medications, then they're not *compliant* with the medications, and then the medications don't *work*. That's why we should focus on patient education."

Corbin was seven years younger than me, but he seemed wise beyond his years. He told me later that he loved hearing my story that day at lunch. But that poker face of his! It disguised all the warmth and empathy I learned to recognize from him years later. I left there thinking, "Does he like me? Does he think this is a good idea? Will he want to work with me?" I had no idea if I'd made a good impression.

But we agreed to meet again. That seemed positive, at least.

A few weeks later, I met him at his office and took a seat in front of his desk. He folded his hands and leaned forward. "Let's work together," he said.

"What?" I asked—almost in disbelief.

He began sketching diagrams on a piece of paper to illustrate how the ideas could work. "Life sciences, biotech, the pharmaceutical industry—all of us need to do better. We need to actually support the patient. I think we could do great things together for patients and their families."

"Yes!" I said excitedly.

"If we really want to move the needle, we should focus on adding value to the patient's life. We should feature real patients, so that other people who share that diagnosis can see themselves in those stories, see hope on the horizon."

My jaw dropped open. Carefully, I closed it and mustered up my courage. "I think I can build this with your help."

"I think you can, too," he said thoughtfully. "Let me think about what that would look like."

Several days later, he called. "I'd like to offer you a consultancy job. We want you to bring your vision for supporting patients to life."

"Expand the patient storytelling approach?!" I asked, elated.

"Exactly. Go find fifty more Brendas."

"I already know the fifty Brendas!" I said gleefully. "I've been meeting people in the MS world for four or five years."

I felt so validated having this smart businessman treating me like an equal. "And—can we have a real patient advisory board?" I asked. I peppered him with questions. "Like, can we work with people from all over the country? Can we take their photos? Can they share their stories? And can we do educational programs all over the country talking about lifestyle, mental health, how they live, and what they do for their MS?"

"Yes. I believe we can," Corbin said calmly. "Build your Patient Ambassador program. Go for it."

A few months later, Corbin and I met at a restaurant to talk more about the Patient Ambassador program. He grabbed a cocktail napkin and took a pen out of his jacket. He was writing something on the napkin. I was starting to learn this was a thing with Corbin—he's always sketching pictures and graphs and visuals everywhere. He finished writing and pushed the napkin toward me. *You need to go start a business*, he'd written.

I looked at him, surprised. "I was thinking about it."

"Do it," he said, nodding.

"So, then I won't be a consultant. You'd be hiring my company?"

"Exactly," he said.

And that was how Snow Companies began. Years later, Corbin joined me as my business partner, along with some of the other amazing people I first met through Serono, Nadine McGowan and Mike Simone.

That was the beginning of a new business—but it signified more than that. It was me taking a crucial step forward in my Patient's Journey: allowing my experiences with navigating MS to propel me into new purpose. I was actively rebuilding my life. I wasn't going to let my disease hinder me from doing important work; in fact, my disease was going to help steer me toward this new mission.

What was my mission? To help a whole lot more patients.

TIME TO REBUILD

It amazes me how many patients I see making big life changes in the Rebuilding phase.

On the other side of their diagnosis, patients feel they've been given the ultimate second chance, the ultimate do-over. You've gone through a season where life-as-you-know-it has been rocked to its core. Everything you were hoping, dreaming, and planning has cracks in it. And in the midst of all that breakage, as you gather knowledge about what is *really* true and meaningful and important, you get greater clarity on what really matters to you. I've seen this more times than I can count; people who have been diagnosed with chronic and terminal conditions—while having a horrible cross to bear—also come away with a deeper sense of the meaning of life.

By now, most patients have had to pare down a lot of the "extras" they used to spend time worrying about, because they need to conserve energy for the stuff that's actually important. And there's a lot of freedom and empowerment when you don't have to do the shit that society tries to impose on you. Who cares about keeping up with the Joneses anymore? You can block out the excess noise. You're *only* putting things into your life that bring you joy, and add value, and are worth it to you.

That can prompt many patients to completely rethink how they spend their time. Those patients who can still work and choose to may change careers. Some people stop working but start devoting some of their limited energy to volunteering or philanthropy. Some people go back to school to pursue a field of study they always wanted to learn about.

In the same way that I changed careers, I've seen many other patients who were able to continue in the workforce completely reinvent their career pursuits. I've seen others leave the workforce altogether to spend their limited time and energy on driving change in areas that matter to them. Some patients become philanthropy rainmakers, helping those in even worse condition than they're in. I've seen people go back to school when they thought they never could or would never want to. I've seen people try things that had always felt off limits because their parents had told them, "You won't be successful at that," or, "You won't make any money." One woman I know was a corporate HR Director who, in the Rebuilding stage of her Patient's Journey, decided she was going to quit all that and become an artist. She had always wanted to be one, and she finally felt the freedom to execute the ultimate reinvention of herself.

In the Rebuilding stage, many patients feel freedom to execute the ultimate reinvention of themselves.

As I've listened to patients share their stories over the years, I've seen that—for many—the Rebuilding phase almost takes on a spiritual quality. You're naturally asking the Big Questions: What do I want my life to be about for as long as I'm still here? What really matters? What do I believe in? How do I want to be remembered? And, as you're asking those questions, you're also dealing with a former life that is now largely in pieces. Your former career might be kaput. Your relationships may have gone through some upheaval. Your own priorities and abilities have changed. So, the combination of that disruption with a revitalized sense of purpose leads many patients to a stunning process of reinvention.

These are some of the gifts of settling into your new normal. All of the work you've done in the Endurance, Optimize Your Relationships, and Optimize Your Care stages begins to pay off. Through making countless deliberate decisions, you have engineered a life that gets you the most stability and energy possible in your life with disease. That opens you up to rebuilding the life you want—the life that will maximize all your remaining minutes.

PATIENT PERSPECTIVE:
TOBIAS W., WISKOTT-ALDRICH SYNDROME

One of my earliest memories is the moment when I learned I was about to die. "He won't live past his tenth birthday," the doctors told my mom, with me sitting right there. The rare disease they had just diagnosed me with, Wiskott-Aldrich Syndrome (WAS), was going to cost me my life, sooner rather than later. From a young age, it struck fear in me.

Since I knew my life had an expiry date, the health consequences of my activities did not concern me. I did everything the other boys my age did, regardless of the injuries I sustained due to WAS. I acted as if I didn't care, but there was no getting away from the emotional cost my condition imposed. When "my time was up," at about ten years of age, I had my first panic attack. As I grew older, I became rebellious, called shady people my friends and had several run-ins with police. I believed I was going to die any day—so why not live recklessly? Drugs and false friends took me on a speedway toward total disaster. In my teens, the doctors started to change their tune, giving me maybe up to twenty years. But the emotional damage of my destructive lifestyle—living under the shadow of death—had already been done. I was alive, but I had no hope.

I came to a new physician who was at the cutting edge of WAS research. He shared spectacular news with me: there was in fact a good chance I could reach retirement age. All of a sudden, I was gifted a life?! But the good news also filled me with horror. What had I done to myself? During one particularly long hospital stay I came to the realization that my behavior had to change drastically. I started proper care, went back to school, and started a career. I met my wife, who gave me courage and hope. She didn't judge me for my difficult past. She also stood by my side when a renewed panic attack presented a major setback. Today we have three wonderful kids who we support on their path to becoming happy people with meaningful lives.

For a long time, I wasn't sure if life was worth living. But as I started to build a life and finally live it, I learned that it is absolutely worth it. We all deserve a chance at building and rebuilding our lives. But that chance may not always be handed to us. Sometimes we have to be vulnerable and ask for help. Sometimes we have to share our fears. Do it! Because I can tell you firsthand: life is precious and worth living, for as long as it lasts.

YOU ARE IN CHARGE OF MAKING YOUR MOMENTS

Rebuild the life you want. Here's why this matters so much: you know by now that life is made up of invaluable minutes you don't get back. As you wake up to your own vulnerability and reckon with your mortality, you start to see life with deeper meaning. Even if you don't have a terminal condition, you get choosy with how you spend your time. These are invaluable minutes you won't get back.

Get choosy with how you spend your time.

In previous chapters, I talked about what to cut *out* to make the most of your limited energy and time: Stupid chores. Annoying people. We talked about how to delegate tasks.

But now, I want to talk about what to fold *in*. I can sum it up in a word: FUN. "Fun" for a lot of people encapsulates joy, happiness, compassion, purpose, and hope—but for me, the word "fun" is synonymous with my mom. It was the memories with my mom that guided me forward into my next stage in the Patient's Journey.

Just as my dad indoctrinated me with the gospel of positivity, my mom raised me on fun. She was an actress, dancer, and fashion queen. For as long as I can remember, our attic was filled with costumes, and on any given day, she would say, "Let's go get the costume box!" We didn't have to choose just one costume for Halloween; we could be four different things, changing along our trick or treating route. And there was no need to buy anything either because we had amassed a huge collection of costume items in the attic, just by gathering things we found. A purple ribbon off a birthday present went in the costume box, and then next thing you knew, it was a hair ribbon and you were a princess.

And, like moths to a flame, people were attracted to her orbit. Mom made sure my sister and I always knew that *every day was going to be fun*. Even when our family didn't have any money, Mom would turn a meager lunch into a picnic on our front lawn, and we'd drink water from fancy glasses and pretend we were fine ladies. We "traveled" in our imagination, too. I had a globe in my room. Mom would often invite me to spin the globe with my eyes closed, and I'd point my finger, stick it on a spot, and we'd look at where it had landed. Then, we'd run together to look up the place in the Encyclopedia Britannica to see what that place was like. I just loved that.

My mother could literally come up with a holiday for every single day of the year. She would find a reason to celebrate 365 days of the year: It's a half-birthday! It's an early Thanksgiving! It's the first day of Spring! It's brownies-with-ice cream day!

I had such a gift in my mother. She gave me the ability to have a creative imagination, which was a game changer when I did visualization exercises to help me get stronger during my early days of MS. But she also instilled in me this vital truth: *you* are in charge of making your moments.

You are in charge of making your moments.

Opportunities don't just fall out of the sky onto your lap. If you want to make memories with your people, or laugh, or celebrate, *you* are in charge of making that happen. Those celebrations don't have to be elaborate or fancy or expensive. But they're yours to make. My mother would have said this years before I ever did: be your own advocate. No one will care about you the way that you will care about you. No one will hand you the answers on a silver platter or create your perfect utopia. So, if you're not going to be a participant or at least be willing to be in the driver's seat at least 50 percent of the time, then you can't really bitch about life being a drag.

Who wants to bitch about anything? Better to have fun instead.

Fun and joy and purpose are all still available to you. Yes, you have physical challenges, and you may have financial hardships as well. But you can still eat dinner on your front lawn on the first warm day of the year, and that can be just as special as if you were dining al fresco in the south of France.

So, let me acquaint you with some of the many ways you can make memorable moments with the time you still have. All of them in some way boil down to this: discover what matters to you, and do it. Do it now rather than later.

Discover what matters to you, and do it. Do it now rather than later.

Architect Normalcy

In the last chapter, we talked about your healthcare plan. We talked about your communication plan. You've got a household management plan. You have the "in case I die or become incapacitated" plan. Lots of plans.

You need one more plan. You need the "What Am I Going to Do *to Still Have Fun?*" plan. And this one is just as important as the others!

Your fun plan doesn't need to be expensive; it just needs to be deliberate. While on this Patient's Journey, you have to *architect normalcy.* You don't want to lose the things that define who you are as a person, or as a couple, or as a family—but it won't be as easy as it might have been before to do them. That's why you need to get creative and plan ahead.

It's easy enough to come up with an *intention,* but you also have to have a plan for execution. For instance, a few years ago, I finally made a plan to lose the extra weight I'd gained during that taco-inhaling steroids season. For years, I'd been *saying,* "I'm going to lose weight, I'm going to lose weight," but—although I had an intention—I never did anything about it. A few years ago, I finally made a plan to execute. Architecting normalcy first begins with your *ideas* of how that might look; then, once you have that idea, put pen to paper and start planning.

There's a lot about returning to normalcy that should become rote: lather, rinse, and repeat. That's true especially if you're newly on this journey and coming out of a lengthy time of intense health challenges. For me, architecting normalcy meant being able to get up before Stephanie, get myself dressed, make her lunch, and get her off to school. That meant getting up extra early, so I had sufficient time to get dressed, which also meant getting to bed early. It meant using my claw-grabber tool to make her lunch. And then, after dropping her off, I had to schedule a ninety-minute nap to recover. I figured out systems to hit each benchmark until that morning routine felt like "lather, rinse, repeat." Once I was able to consistently show up for those nonnegotiables, *then* I was able to add in the extra fun stuff: travel, getting back to work, building a platform, volunteering, and so on.

Everything needs to be done via baby steps. Go slow. Be kind to yourself. Your health challenges most likely progressed for a while. Likewise, your new normal won't suddenly spring into place. It will take some time to get your footing and feel out what that will look like for you.

You don't want to lose the things that define who you are as a person, but doing them won't be as easy as it may have been before. Get creative and plan ahead to architect normalcy and fun.

Other areas of your life may simply look different in this new normal—and that's okay. Every chronic illness has with it particular areas that are more challenging in terms of your unique health deficits. For example, when Stephanie was young, I was not the parent who could stand on the sidelines of her soccer games for an hour, or go to games on days when it was extremely hot. I couldn't attend the early morning games. But I also learned a few hacks to help me show up whenever possible. I traveled with a camping chair that was easy to set up, so that I could sit down when most people would be comfortable standing. I got a cooling vest early on to help keep my core temperature down, so I had more flexibility on hot days. Gradually, through planning and finding those little hacks, I expanded the "normalcy" and fun I could return to.

Here's the good news: there are new gadgets and devices coming on the market all the time. If you devote a good afternoon to some Google searching, you're likely to find all sorts of hacks and tools that will help you relaunch yourself back into society.

So, consider: How can you still do things that bring your family joy, even in the midst of illness? Enough of your life will be altered and sad. This is not the time to give up *everything*. This is the time to hang on like hell to the stuff that brings you joy. Look for the creative work-arounds to make participation possible, so that you can architect normalcy and joy into your life.

This is the time to hang on like hell to the stuff that brings you joy.

"Travel"

Remember my mom's spinning globe vacations? You can do the same thing with Google Earth. If you're facing a long day in the hospital or in your bed, pull out your smartphone or tablet and ask your care partner, "Where do we want to travel today?" You can virtually go there! In fact, you can see places on Google Earth that you could never travel to, even when healthy.

The internet has opened up opportunities that can connect you with people from all over the world. This is especially valuable if you have a rare disease and there are only a few thousand people with the same condition. You can connect with those people even if they're in a different country. (Remember the site www.patientworthy.com, a site that helps patients with rare diseases find each other.) Those connections can be a powerful way to find support for your unique disease and remember you're not alone.

There's a cautionary piece to this too, though: real living requires real human connection. As much as possible (extreme pandemic conditions excepted), you don't want to be so isolated that your only interactions are through a computer screen. Everything that makes a screen or the internet great can also become a drain on your life if it becomes all that you're doing, ten hours a day.

Travel to real places, if you can. I know a patient who saves a dollar a day for vacations, and gradually increases the amount throughout the year. During January, every day, a dollar goes into an envelope. In February, it's two dollars per day. In March, it's three, and so on. By the time they get to the end of the year, they've saved up over two thousand dollars. That's been a method that has worked for them, even when they were on a limited budget. Their kids contributed to the family vacation bank too, and it was something they did together every year—as a family and as a team.

You want to go to Disney World? Do it! And research ahead of time how it's going to work to get around in a wheelchair. (Psst:

they let you cut to the front of the lines!) Do you still want to do the family camping trip? Good! How can you get creative to work out those logistics? Are you immunocompromised and don't want to fly on a plane? You still have options! Plan to rent an RV, make this The Year of the Road Trip, and go to a few National Parks.

Connect with human beings in real life if you can. And when you can't, lean on technology for creative ways to "travel" and connect with others.

Embrace Humor

For me, it's been a lifeline in the midst of my disease to maintain a sense of humor and even enjoy the irony of awkward situations. For example, once, I was preparing to give a keynote address to a big pharma company. This was a large event, so I had gotten a wireless mic clipped on my shirt. As an MS patient, I have dicey bladder control, so I always go to the bathroom right before a speech, just to tick the box.

I asked the sound engineer, "Okay, how much time before I go on?"

"Five minutes," he whispered.

"Great, I'm going to use the bathroom," I whispered back. I went, peed, flushed, and washed my hands. Then I came back out.

Everyone backstage was *looking* at me. And the sound engineer was *looking* at me—with sort of a shocked, aghast expression. "What's going on?" I asked the sound engineer.

He said, "I'm sorry—you were on a hot mic."

I paused. "You mean *everybody* heard me go to the bathroom?" I looked out at the hundreds of people in the audience. "This whole fucking room?"

He nodded. "Yeah. Everybody heard."

"Well," I said. "Shit." Then I thought, *Thank God I didn't shit! And thank God I washed my hands.*

That's when the event manager said, "Brenda! You're on."

As I walked to the main stage, feeling super nervous and horribly embarrassed, I thought, *I've got two ways to play this. I can either give my speech feeling distracted and mortified about what people think of me the whole time. Or, I can go up and make a joke about this.*

So, I walked up and said, "My name is Brenda Snow. I know that you all know me because of my role in the MS community. But I think you *really* know me now, because we all just went to the bathroom together!" Everybody laughed. I said, "So, now that we can put that aside, let's get started."

Humor has been a lifeline for me in the midst of my disease and even enables me to enjoy the irony of awkward situations.

How many times has my MS gotten me into embarrassing situations? Too many to count. I've had to use my sense of humor not only to cope with the embarrassing symptoms but also to adjust and adapt to situations when I knew my disease could set me up for awkwardness. I try to get ahead of it by making a joke.

None of us get to live with guarantees. We're not assured of anything. But despite that, our tendency when we get sick is to go, "Why me? Why did this happen to me?" And, as I've discussed, that attitude can keep you stuck. Humor, for me, breaks me out of that. I've said before, "Well, why *not* me? I'm no better or different than anyone else with a disease." On hard days, I try to find funny things to pull me out of a bad mood. Even when the Asshole Doctor came by my rehab room (right before I cussed him out), I was able to reframe that later through humor: he looked like the Man with the Yellow Hat, from *Curious George*. I was so angry, but that thought made me laugh.

Humor will prevent the heavy, dark emotions from eating away at your soul. It adds levity and lightens the burden so that the cross you bear doesn't feel quite so intense. It's a balancing act, of course— plenty of times, the situation is grave and serious and needs your full attention. But other times, your self-deprecating humor can help you embrace the irony in awkward situations and put your companions at ease.

In a weird way, it's also a strategy that helps you take back control. That doesn't necessarily happen on a conscious level—I never woke up and said, "I'm going to use humor today to take back control." But because I maintained a sense of humor and tried, even in the darkest times, to find ways to have fun, those choices to laugh were like little building blocks. They all went into my toolkit to help me navigate my disease. On the really bad days, when I got terrible news—those humor tools were there. They made things just a little easier.

Find Your Village

It's also important to establish a network of people who "get it." It's a gift to have friends who understand what you're going through, who you can be vulnerable with and connected to.

I used to be the type of person who liked my home to look a certain way. If I hadn't made it *just so* with the flowers on the table and the right food in the oven and the perfect champagne, you couldn't come over. It just wasn't going to be that way.

After MS, it was a different story. I once had some close friends over, and one of them asked, "What's this?" She was pointing to something on the floor of the hallway between the kitchen and the bedroom. It was a pair of dirty underwear.

I said, "Well, I guess it's our dirty clothes on the floor." And then we both just laughed.

I consider that moment a little win. I would rather have people over who are comfortable with my new normal and still be accepted than strive for self-imposed perfection. I've often said over the years that sometimes I think it's only Type A people who get a chronic condition, because it's the universe's way of forcing us to chill out a little!

So, try to find people you can laugh with. You can call them your village, your soul people, your besties, your community—but that group of people is going to be an important element of you rebuilding your life toward purpose and fun. And as I've said before, curating your community might mean you say goodbye to some people in your life that aren't able to work with your new normal. That can be hard to do.

Still: it's important to have a network of people that you can be yourself with. You want people who will laugh at your story about a hot mic, or your joke about cutting off your tits; you want people who will see your sign on your walker that says, "Fuck cancer," and say, "This is great, I love this!" Life is too short to be anything other than your authentic self.

Try to find people you can laugh with. Life is too short to be anything other than your authentic self.

Where do you find these people? I've given you some sugges-
tions in other chapters, but keep in mind, your own self-advocacy
will go a long way in helping you connect with them. Remember
the internet is a tool to help you connect with other patients who
might be in your same boat. And remember that, sometimes, you
have to be brave enough to take the first step by joining a support
group or reaching out to a friend you've lost touch with. You might
elect to join a local hobby base to be around non-sick people who
help you remember how to do the things you love. These friends
who "get it" will help buoy you on days when you need a good
laugh or simply an understanding friend.

Celebrate the Wins

Whenever you manage to successfully architect normalcy and find
ways to continue doing the things you love, register that. Celebrate
it! For example, a good friend of mine is supporting her dad who
is dealing with the one-two punch of getting diagnosed with pros-
tate cancer shortly after he got diagnosed with Parkinson's. He was
already adjusting to life with Parkinson's. Now he's going through
radiation and chemo on top of it. Basically, nothing seems great
right now.

My friend has told me how her dad has always been an athlete.
He *lives* for sports. He's not able to participate in sports himself
right now because of what's happening to him physically, but she
makes sure he's able to go to every one of her kids' soccer games.
He's able to watch from the sidelines and still experience the sense
of joy that athletics brings him.

It might take a community to help raise you up and facilitate
those moments that bring back fun. But if and when you make them

happen, those little wins are a game changer. Early in my diagnosis, when I was still moving through the stages of Grief and Anger and Acceptance, the little wins for me were discovering I could do something that, for a time, I hadn't been able to do. For example, before I was diagnosed, I loved going to the pool with Stephanie in the summertime. After developing heat sensitivity with MS, I had to look for ways I could still have a day at the pool with my daughter. When I finally got us back there, swim sessions weren't half a day; they looked more like ninety minutes or maybe two hours. I sat in the shade the whole time and had one of those spray bottle fans—but we got our pool time. And that was a little win.

Any time you find yourself having self-limiting doubt—"I can't do that anymore"—push that aside. Look for creative work-arounds. You may not be able to do the things you love in the same manner you did them before, but almost always, there are ways you can enjoy them in a different capacity. You have too much life left to live to self-limit.

You have too much life left to live to self-limit.

Push yourself to try the things that you didn't expect yourself to be able to do anymore. And when you do it, count it as a win.

Don't Limit Your Options

I could sum all this up by telling you to say "yes" to yes. Don't limit your options. Don't assume, just because you're sick, you can't do things anymore. Give yourself permission to have fun and say *"yes"* to possibilities.

That's easier than you think. Once your community adjusts to
you living with disease, a lot of people will invite you to do stuff
with them. If you've been trained to accept or decline an invitation,
your inclination might be to say no because you don't know how
you're going to feel on that day. But instead, try giving a conditional
yes. I recommend you be honest and ask for permission to give them
late notice: "Can I tell you on Friday if I feel like I can go?" And if
you're up for it on Friday, go! And if you're not, send them a text
and explain you're just feeling too ill to make it.

Even if it's last minute, don't feel like you're being rude. People
will get it. (Remember how your community is slowly going to be
curated so that it's made up of people who get it?) They love you
and understand what you're going through.

This same approach applies to the bigger category of professional
or volunteer work. The whole point of this book is to help you rebuild
without limits. Would you like to go back to work, either full time
or part time? Would you like to start an entirely new career because
the job you used to do is no longer realistic or appealing? Do you
want to find other ways to add value to society? What sounds good
to you? Don't put limits on yourself in pursuing it!

Yes, there may be some hurdles to get over and once again, your
honesty will be required. For instance, if you choose to return to
your former job, you may need to have some courageous conversations with your employer and team members about setting up
accommodations. You may also have to send deliberate cues to your
work or volunteer community about how to treat you and show
you respect. It will be important for you to model the empathy and
vulnerability you hope to experience from others: "Look, it's going
to be one of those days where I can only give fifty percent. I'm

committed to delivering at a later date when I'm back to my baseline, and I'm grateful for your patience in the meantime." You will learn how the good days feel, how the bad days feel, and what your boundaries need to be. Lead with candid, authentic honesty to facilitate understanding; most people will respond to you in kind.

If you know that work is no longer something that makes sense for you, consider volunteering. There is so much need in today's society! If the volunteer side excites you, who *better* to serve others than someone with a chronic illness? You have enormous empathy, insight, and compassion to share as a result of going through this Patient's Journey. Over thirty years into my diagnosis, I've shown up to volunteer or share my story countless times; sometimes, I forget that the collective experience I bring to the table is unique. When I see lightbulbs go on for people—"Oh my goodness, I didn't know this"—I'll realize with surprise that *I* shined a bit of light in that moment.

So, don't let the fear of judgment stop you from entering back into humanitarian work or any kind of career you want to do. Only you, by putting limits on yourself and thinking, "I *can't* do _____" rather than "I *can* do _____" will be the barrier to expanding your options. Your world will become very small, very quickly if you assume all possibilities are now void for you. They're not. So, say "yes" to yes!

Don't limit your options. Say "yes" to yes!

MESSAGE TO CARE PARTNERS: YOUR REBUILDING

Just like your loved one must focus not on what they've lost but on what they *can* and *want* to do, you may also choose to reinvent your life along the new parameters. Listen: you don't have to wait until you have a diagnosis of your own to ask yourself the Big Questions! What really matters to you? You get to reinvent in this season as well. Ask and answer those questions, then start doing things to get what you really want to get out of this life.

As you explore some of your own new dreams and goals, have a conversation with your loved one about how you can explore those in tandem. Try to include them in your dreams. Here's the thing: if you plan to maintain a committed relationship with your loved one, your new normal *will* be different from your old normal. Architecting normalcy doesn't necessarily mean everything goes back to the way it was before your loved one's diagnosis. It means *elements* of that old life return, with adjustments. The sooner you can accept and embrace your new life hacks, the sooner fun can return.

Perhaps, pre-diagnosis, you and your loved one enjoyed hiking together, or doing extreme sports. You want those hiking experiences again—but if you schedule a bunch of major climbing trips and simply say, "Peace out," to your loved one, the patient may feel resentful and left behind. Instead, have a conversation about how you can still enjoy those activities together. Maybe you find hikes that are shorter and mostly level, ones that you can do together. The two of you might get hooked on an extreme sports show you both enjoy watching, or perhaps your loved one cheers you on from the finish line as you complete a triathlon.

Find ways to do the things you love *that still include* the patient in your life. Does that mean you never do the big hikes you love most? No—perhaps you schedule those trips with friends every so often. But you also invest time and effort into including your loved one in your dreams, as much as possible.

If the journey for one person in a couple changes, the journey for the couple must also change. If you as a care partner can't abide those changes, your shared trajectory will become bifurcated. Staying together means aligning what you do as a unit. Find ways to cultivate and architect the experiences that strengthen your connection and bring you both joy.

BRAS AND SWAMP COOLERS IN THE HARRY POTTER ATTIC

A few years after I started Snow Companies, we had two clients on board with steadily growing work. Slowly, we were getting traction. I had just made the nerve-racking leap to hire a third person for my team, and now we needed to find an office space. But I didn't just want any old office space—I wanted to be *home,* so that I could be there for Stephanie when she got home from school.

"Home," by now, was Virginia. In my travels around the country, I'd spoken to an MS support group in Virginia and was struck by how beautiful it was. I did some digging and found out there were many areas with incredible public education. The houses were affordable and huge, compared to my tiny California bungalow. And my visit was in the spring, when Virginia was sunny, lush, and temperate.

As a disabled, broke California girl, I was eager to find a place where I could afford a better life for Stephanie. I did the math and realized that if I sold my house in California, I could pay off most of my remaining medical debt and still have enough to move to Virginia and buy the type of home that I would *never* be able to afford in California. *What else can I lose?* I thought. *Why not?* We packed our bags, said goodbye to our family on the West Coast, and moved into a classic brick colonial in a tranquil Williamsburg neighborhood. It had four bedrooms, three baths, a half-acre lot, and cost a third of what I got from selling my California house. *Surely, we can squeeze an office for Snow Companies into my great big house,* I thought. That would certainly be the cheapest thing. The third-floor attic was a small space—not much bigger than Harry Potter's closet under the stairs at the Dursley's. But it would do! So, I scraped up all the savings I had at that point in my life, which was right around $8,000, and called a contractor. The contractor I liked best quoted me $12,000 to do the job.

"I can only spend $7,000," I informed him. "What can you do to bring it down to $7,000?"

He sighed and pushed a hand through his hair, studying the small attic space. "We could pull the air conditioning lines," he said. "That's a big expense."

That sounded like a problem. Despite my first impression of Virginia in the fragrant, mild spring, I had learned that my new hometown got hot as Hades in the summer, and I was extra sensitive to heat. The attic was already hot and stuffy. "How else could we air it?" I asked.

He said, "For $7,000, we can put one of those swamp coolers in the wall. We'd leave access to the back, and you'd have to periodically drain a bucket of water to keep it running cool. But that would kind of cool this place down."

I didn't know what the hell he was talking about, but I was like, "Okay, if that's what we can afford, we'll take it."

He agreed. "I've got a project going for the rest of July," he said. "I can get you all set up, come August."

So, for all of July, my two team members and I tried working up there. We were *dying* in that heat. We sat in that small space, under the sloping ceilings, typing away at our laptops with sweat pouring down our foreheads. One of them, Meredith, spoke with this beautiful Southern drawl, and she said, "Gawd *dayem,* it's hot in heah."

I said, "Yes. It is *so* hot. I'm sweating through my clothes." Then I said, "I can't take it anymore. I'm sorry, but I have to make things awkward." I stripped off my shirt and went back to typing in my bra, grateful that at that point, we were an all-girl team.

The other two women looked at each other. Then, Meredith stripped off her shirt, too. The other woman followed suit.

I wondered, *Are these women* actually *so hot that they need to do this, or are they just trying to make me feel better because of my MS?* Either way, it was amazing to have that kind of support, because there was no way I could sit up in that attic in proper work attire.

Thank God it was the pre-Zoom era!

Talk about friends that "get it"—those women were amazing team members. We laughed every day. And until the damn swamp cooler had been installed, we all worked in various stages of undress.

As Snow Companies gradually got bigger and bigger over the years, I still tried to find ways to inject silliness and fun into the mix. There was no more stripping down (thank God), but there has been lots of dressing up. Our Halloween parties are epic—a legacy I have inherited from my mother, the Queen of Fun. We time our Snow Companies party with a blood drive, so we're giving back at the same time we're embracing our inner kids. The different teams at Snow all plan themed costumes, and everyone goes next level. Our 40,000 square foot office space (quite a difference from the attic where we started!) gets completely transformed. Last year, one team transformed their area into Hogwarts. Another team did *Game of Thrones*. Another one did Mario Kart, and you could sit on a skateboard and drive yourself through the building. It's just *fun*. I want my team to know that, even while I take the business seriously and I take my MS seriously, I also want to be a role model of a person who lives with humor, positivity, and approachability. I want to be remembered as someone who embraced *fun*.

Whether we're dealing with illness, or work, or anything else—there are always high stakes. Yes, these things matter, and we need to take them seriously. But that doesn't mean we need to be serious *all the time*.

There are always high stakes. But that doesn't mean we need to be serious *all the time*.

You deserve to make every second count. Remember: these are invaluable minutes you don't get back! So, be discerning about the company you keep and don't have such a fatalistic attitude. In the Rebuilding phase of the Patient's Journey, the most incredible blessings can come.

Look for them. Celebrate them! Laugh as often as you can and look for ways to architect fun and normalcy. And as all these little wins build up, you'll remember that life on the other side of disease can still be so, so rich.

From that place of renewal, you're ready for the final stage in your Patient's Journey: Impact.

STAGE 9 OF THE PATIENT'S JOURNEY: REBUILDING

- *Common emotions: increased energy and creativity, motivation to (re)engage in new or familiar contexts, inspiration over possible forms of investment, eagerness to find solutions and work-arounds to architect normalcy.*

- *Common pitfalls: a "can't do it" attitude, resentment toward care partner for their comparative ease of living, getting overwhelmed by the challenges of building back normalcy.*

- *Your best next step: Carpe diem! These are invaluable minutes you don't get back. As you regain energy and learn how to manage your symptoms, be proactive about architecting fun and normalcy back into your life.*

CHAPTER 11

Impact

YOUR STORY IS A GIFT TO THOSE AROUND YOU

"The people who are crazy enough to think they can change the world are the ones who do."

— Steve Jobs

You started this journey gutted and grief-stricken. When you were diagnosed with a chronic or terminal disease, you may have felt suddenly irrelevant. Marginalized. Invisible.

That was the *beginning* of your Patient's Journey. It is not the end.

As you move your way through the Acceptance, Endurance, and Optimize Your Relationships and Care stages, and begin to reinvent yourself in the Rebuilding stage—you're now ready to do something that may have felt impossible at the start of this journey.

You're ready to start helping other people with your story.

You are now uniquely qualified to make an impact on a patient population that is desperate for your encouragement. Yes, you can make an impact because of this disease. You can change lives as a result of navigating this journey!

It is time to start helping other people with your story.

I know the feeling of being marginalized and irrelevant. People didn't used to give me the time of day. I can't tell you how many times I wasn't taken seriously by the corporate world or leaders in the life sciences industry. One of my first meetings took place in a company boardroom shortly after I had started my company. I was looking for new clients, and after I had pitched my idea that biotech companies should tell more patient stories and give patients resources to help them on their journey, one of the men at the table smirked. He said, "That's a cute idea. Did you come up with that all by yourself?"

I had seen these sorts of looks from men before. Even before I got sick, I had experienced men's looks that tried to sum me up in a few words: "Dumb blonde, big tits." Only, with this San Francisco crew, they had the luxury of adding in a special new adjective: "Dumb, *crippled* blonde. Big tits." Clearly, they weren't taking me seriously.

One of the other men at the table said, "Thank you, Ms. Snow, I think we've heard enough." I was hurried out of the boardroom.

Over twenty years after I started telling my story, things have changed.

Snow Companies got a lot of traction early on, especially in the area of multiple sclerosis. Working with our first client, we built services and programs to support people and their families dealing with the diagnosis of MS. In those early days, our focus was on sharing real, authentic patient stories. As a result, we were able to showcase all the things people could do to potentially change the course of their illness, including therapeutics, emotional connection, and hands-on strategies for living a self-determined life with an illness. By sparking positive conversations between patients, their loved ones, and their healthcare providers, patients began to see themselves as people again, not just as patients. They became empowered to reclaim their dignity, knowing that while disease may be a part of them, they are much more than just a syndrome or an interesting medical case. They're human.

Snow Companies became more successful—it was clear we were tapping into patients' unmet needs. I could see that the company had potential to do much more for all the other patients dealing with a life-changing diagnosis. At that point, I decided I didn't want Corbin Wood as a client anymore. He was a fantastic mentor and I wanted him to be my business partner. Thankfully, he agreed to join.

Then, somewhere along the way, Snow Companies turned into a rocket ship.

Every year since 2001, Snow Companies has experienced greater success than the year before. At the time of this writing, we now employ over 400 people, we have active disease awareness campaigns on six continents, we've won countless awards for our short films, we've pioneered using social media platforms for healthcare outreach, and we've helped tens of thousands of Patient Ambassadors share their inspirational stories with millions of people all over the globe. Every year, we get the privilege of talking to more patients and their families. Then, we get to see them go out and change additional people's lives by sharing hope.

That, to me, is the truest indicator of Snow Companies' success. More than the number of employees, the revenue, or any other indicator, I have sought to measure Snow Companies' success by what we're doing for patients. Every day, I asked: Are we standing by them, honoring their stories, and giving them important information? Are we adding meaning and hope to their lives? I sought to hold true to my core tenets and values, to keep us focused on making a positive impact in the world. As I reflect during the writing of this book, I know that's what we've accomplished. Our success is measured by the thousands of letters and emails we've received from patients or their family members, telling us how they were helped by our services and programs, or by hearing a Patient Ambassador's inspirational story.

Every single one of those Patient Ambassadors started their Patient's Journey in the same place you did: Feeling despair. Feeling grief. Wondering if life was over. Experiencing devastating loneliness.

Now, patients like you are changing lives with their stories. Whenever one of them shares their amazing story with an audience of other patients, people are visibly moved. Afterward, audience members come up to them and say things like, "Hearing your story makes me feel like I can keep going."

If you initially felt surprised to see that the final stage in the Patient's Journey is Impact, don't be. I've seen it a million times. *Impact* is where your Journey takes you. It's time to join an army of encouragers.

Yes: there's happiness and joy ahead. Yes: you can even be a role model for others. On the other side of this Journey, you'll have the perspective to share your experiences with others in need—and your story can be the ultimate gift to someone else who needs the hope you can give them to move forward. Do not underestimate the massive power of encouraging someone at their lowest point to keep trying. Your story might be the catalyst that saves someone's life. I'm not speaking hyperbolically—I have seen this and heard this more times than I can count after watching a Patient Ambassador share their story.

You get to change the world.

Impact is where your Journey takes you. Join an army of encouragers and change the world.

RECOGNIZE THE NEED FOR IMPACT

I want you to think for a moment about why you picked up this book. Consider the emotional state you were in when you began reading Chapter 1. What were you looking for? What help did you hope to find here?

I'm guessing your answers fall somewhere in the categories of encouragement, hope, reassurance, or guidance. The longing to know you were not alone.

Now: consider how many hundreds of thousands of other patients and care partners exist in the world whose lives have just been radically altered by illness. Think of how many people will hear a devastating diagnosis, just *today.*

They need hope. They need someone to tell them their lives aren't over. They need a strong hug, and they need someone to say, "I've been through it, and it's going to be okay. It's hard, and there will be a lot of rocky days. But it will get easier. There's still a good life waiting for you."

**Think of how many people will hear a devastating diagnosis, just
today. They need someone to say, "I've been through it, and it's going
to be okay. There's still a good life waiting for you."**

If you have been encouraged or helped at all by this book, or if
you have had a single conversation with another human being
throughout your own Patient's Journey that helped put a smile on
your face and lifted you up—then, you know. You know how great
the need is for the impact that *you* are now equipped to make.

In most of the countless conversations I've had with patients, I
usually find that what they need from me at first is reassurance that
it's going to be okay. Then, they need enthusiasm and motivation
to keep pushing forward on their Journey. They need to know that
they can do this and they've got this.

It takes a lot to muster up the energy to pour that out to others.
And for that reason, I'm thankful for all the grit I had to develop
throughout the prior stages of the Patient's Journey; it's helping me
now. I needed to go through it myself to be able to give. I've honed
the skills to be an empowered patient. I know how to advocate for
myself and others. I've learned how to manage my energy so that I
can spend it where it matters. And I want to spend it impacting
people's lives.

This is where it matters. If you have made it to the Impact stage
of your Patient's Journey, you might be able to see hundreds of other
patients in your rearview mirror: Still struggling with bewilderment
in the Diagnosis stage. Still with their head down in the Grief stage.
Still consumed with rage in the Anger stage. Maybe they've come
to a place of Acceptance of their illness, but they're not yet

convinced they have what it takes to move forward. You might see some making connections and discoveries in the Endurance stage, but they could really use some advice. You might see some contemplating a courageous step in the Rebuilding stage, and they need some cheering on. These patients need you! They need your reassurance, enthusiasm, and motivation to keep going. They need you to help normalize their struggle. They need your tips and tricks that helped you along. They need *your story*. If and when you choose to share your story more broadly, you'll see just how much it can inspire others. People listen to you in tears. You have overcome something you never thought you could, and that's inspiring to people.

When I was lying in the Long-Term Rehab Care facility in 1994, it was an isolating place. It was a neurological rehabilitation floor, which meant most of the patients were well into their seventies and eighties. I just kept looking around and thinking, *God, I'd give* anything *to talk to one person like me*. I didn't want more occupational therapy. I didn't care about getting the best med. I just wanted to talk to *one* person like me. That was it. I wanted someone to say to me, "It's going to be okay."

I didn't ever find that person. But I finally met a physical therapist who specialized in MS who said, "There are other people like you."

"Where *are* they?" I asked. "They're not here!"

She said, "Well, I can't disclose that information. Patient confidentiality. But they're out there. You should try to meet them!"

It was because of that comment that I gathered up the courage to attend a self-help group meeting. I did meet some great people there. However, most of the people I met were in a very negative place and quite advanced in their MS. I was looking for someone to tell me everything would be okay—but no one had *anything* to say. No one even smiled. Even though I'm glad they didn't try to give me false hope, I left feeling really sad and broken.

But the experience also made me realize what I might have to bring to the table: I wanted to bring some positivity. I wanted to put a smile on people's faces. I thought, *There has to be something better than this. You can't tell me there are 400,000 people who have MS in the United States and no one can do any better than this. Somebody out there has to do better than this.*

That thought planted a seed: *maybe that's supposed to be me.*

I didn't know what that impact might look like; I just recognized the need and saw that I wanted to do something about filling it. Years later, when I had the courage to knock on doors and start sharing my story, it was because I wanted to try to take other patients from that sad, broken place I had been, to a place where they felt encouraged and inspired.

I wanted to try to take patients from a sad, broken place,

to encouragement and inspiration.

And that's exactly what happened: every time I have shared my story—fifteen to forty-five minutes of being authentic, sharing real perspectives about living with illness, and ending on a note of positivity—people have been changed. Patients in the audience stand in a line to talk to me, hug me, cry with me.

In the years that I've run Snow, I've seen this same scene play out with countless other Patient Ambassadors. *So* many stories have been shared—from patients dealing with epilepsy, cancer, rheumatoid arthritis, psoriasis, and so on. They talk about their Journey: from the devastated place they began, to the renewed and purpose-filled place they've arrived. People who are earlier in their Journeys are profoundly moved. I hear about it in countless emails and phone calls afterward—I get more than I can handle.

The same transformational shift happens for care partners, too. I can't tell you how many parents I've seen at these events who are caring for their sick kids, and they are so desperate for this encouraging human connection. You can't imagine how impactful it is for these moms to hear another mom share her story of walking alongside her child through illness. They cry with one another and hug; I hear them say, "I have felt like a failure, all this time. What can I do to help? All I want is to be there for my kid."

I've even witnessed this play out internationally. I have watched Patient Ambassadors share their stories all over the world in languages I don't understand, but I can still see the narrative of their Patient Journey play out through their body language and tone of voice. And the impact is universal: their audiences tear up with emotion. They smile and laugh. The energy in the room is uplifting and healing—both for the Patient doing the sharing and all the others doing the listening.

I had always suspected it would be helpful for patients to share their stories with one another, especially if the stories ended in a hopeful place. But even *I* could never have anticipated just how great the need is and just how significant the potential for impact.

Listen: there is *so much power* in sharing what's happened to you. Snow Companies would not have achieved the success it has otherwise. Your Journey through hell, to hope, to greater wholeness is the story that someone else needs.

Your Journey through hell, to hope, to greater wholeness is the story that someone else needs.

Make It Count

My story of becoming the founder and CEO of a large patient engagement company is unique. I'm not suggesting this has to be everybody's path. Your own form of impact will be tailored to your context, timing, available energy, situation, and sense of purpose. And let me just say: as triumphant as I feel about building a global organization, I felt equal triumph on the first day that I was able to get out of bed and make toast for my daughter. I hold that win just as dearly as I hold building Snow Companies, and the latter would have never happened without the former.

Each step mattered. Each win was significant.

So, here's how I want you to frame your own aspirations for impact: *make your moments count*. Don't lose sight of your hopes and dreams; take small steps in their direction. Have an attitude that will keep you open to serendipity. Be okay with embracing the unexpected. Look for ways to impact others in a positive way. And celebrate every single little win along the way.

Also, keep in mind that your illness has opened you to avenues of impact you would have never encountered otherwise! Had I not gotten MS, I never would have built the business I did. I would have been happy in an average career, plugging along, doing my thing.

But because I got MS, I discovered a passion to help other patients. I developed the fortitude I needed to get it started. I developed the stick-to-it-iveness to see it through. Granted, I also benefited from good luck, having the right people on my team, and I've put in a lot of hard work. But at the end of the day, the reason Snow Companies happened is because I was trying to fix *me*. I was trying to find a way to make this shit okay.

Your own efforts toward impact don't need to be purely altruistic—you can be just as selfish as I was. Helping others is a huge mood boost for yourself. It helps validate all the hell you've had to push through! Your impact can and *should* benefit you, in small and large ways. I know many other patients with chronic or terminal illnesses that have built thriving businesses. I know people who have built amazing philanthropic initiatives. I know patients who have families that are absolutely thriving because they chose to stay home and put their energy there. And whenever patients invest in others, something almost magical seems to happen: they feel better in body, heart, and soul.

When you find ways to invest in others, that impact makes illness easier to bear. You realize helping others actually helps *you*. Given your limits and available energy, what is something you can do to leave the world just a little bit better than how you found it?

So, consider: What is going to be your thing? The magnitude doesn't matter; you're simply looking for the best place to put your energy. How do you want to spend your time? How *can* you spend your time? Given your limits and available energy, what is something you can do to leave the world just a little bit better than how you found it?

I've seen patients pursue forms of impact in any number of ways—here are just a few examples:

- Volunteering with a cause close to their heart
- Joining a political committee or civic organization
- Counseling traumatized people with the empathy and insights they gained through navigating their illness
- Helping children learn to read through participating in a literacy program
- Taking on physical challenges that, during the lowest lows of their illness, would have seemed impossible
- Returning to their old career
- Starting a new career

There's no right or wrong about how you pursue making a positive difference; there's only what's right for your Journey.

PATIENT PERSPECTIVE: CARRIE S., MS

After I was diagnosed, everything seemed so dark and uncertain. I remember my mom saying to me in the midst of this nightmare, "One day you will use this story as a testimony." At the time, it really aggravated me. I was unreceptive to that thought. I didn't *want* a testimony—I wanted my old life back. I wanted my health back. I wanted to be able to take care of my daughter. I wanted to sing and play music again. My life had turned to ashes and I didn't know how to move forward.

Since I had a child that was depending on me, I didn't have the option to "check out" on life. I had to power through. I had to move on. But then the question became: *How* do I do that? I had to realize that this was just a chapter of my life—not the whole book. The words of my mom kept playing in my head and the answer came loud and clear: stop focusing on yourself and start helping others! I decided that I would try to serve others using the medium I knew best: my music. I wrote a song about my experience and shared that, along with my story, to thousands of patients and caregivers. I saw lives and attitudes changed through that song. In my experience, music can touch the heart where mere words fail. It can transform one's outlook. It can uplift and inspire. As I was able to touch others' lives, I saw the transformation happening in my own life. When I stopped focusing on *me* and my own troubles, I saw real changes taking place.

The blessing of my support network, my family, my husband, and my daughter, was also a huge reason I found strength to give back. Playing an active part in my daughter's life and watching her grow into the most amazing human being that I know has had a profound impact on my attitude. Being able to share my story with others and getting back to being a mom, wife, and musician—those are the things that pulled me out of the ashes. As I focused on these amazing points of impact, suddenly I noticed that the ashes had turned to gold. I was finally moving on to the next chapter of my life, and what an inspiring chapter it has been!

SHARE YOUR STORY

In whatever context you choose for Impact—whether that's in the professional world; in philanthropy; among friends, family, church groups, or other patients—let me ask you to do one thing: share your story.

If you look at the history of humanity, back to the days when early humans were drawing pictures on walls, you find stories. Humans have a rich "Oral History" for a reason. Enslaved peoples told each other stories of their ancestors. People who didn't have the ability to read or write often sang songs about their story. From the time language was invented, stories have been used to convey values, lessons, or memories.

I don't know how many people will ever say, "I watched a fifty-two slide PowerPoint presentation today that changed my life." Fuck no. But you will hear any number of people say, "I heard the most amazing *story* today."

"I met this incredible Patient Ambassador today. She changed my life."

"Hearing *your story* gives me hope to keep going."

I've experienced it. I've witnessed it thousands of times for other Patient Ambassadors. And being partly responsible for all those moments is an honor I hold profoundly dear.

If you're reading this book, I hope you are inspired with this takeaway: write your story.

It doesn't have to be hundreds of pages. When we assist patients in writing their stories, we usually shoot for 1,500 words or less. It might take fifteen minutes to share and will keep the audience engaged, hitting on all the important points while leaving out tangential information. Of course, it can be longer if you want—there's no right or wrong.

How do you start? I recommend writing a letter to your younger self. Think about who you were at the start of your Patient's Journey, and consider the following prompts:

- Validate the tough spot you were in during that low point in your life. Relate to your younger self to demonstrate that you haven't forgotten how difficult it was. Describe the sights, sounds, and smells of the place you were in. Describe the fears that haunted you.
- Share some of the life lessons you've learned through this Journey.
- Note some of the things you're amazed you've overcome.
- Help your younger self by expressing some of the key truths you know now that you didn't know at the start of your Journey.

Start there, and write a basic, two-page letter. You will be amazed how much beauty and wisdom comes just from responding to those few prompts.

At the very least, this exercise will be profoundly beneficial for you. I've worked with many patients who really *went there* with this letter writing exercise and got vulnerable. Afterwards, they told me, "I'm not ready to share this with anyone." That's okay—just because you write it doesn't mean you have to share it. But simply writing the letter will help you tap into some inner strength that you didn't even know you had. You will reflect and think to yourself, *Actually—I've done a pretty damn good job*, or, *I didn't think about that.*

At most, your story has the power to help many, many other people. If you decide you want to expand that letter into a fuller story to share with others, add in the broader context of your Patient's Journey. When I share my own story, I start by painting the picture of what I looked like thirty years ago. I give them an idea of just how bad my MS was, and I give them a look into my life as a mom. I'm transparent about the lows: how poor we were, my various levels of being handicapped, and all the different moments of struggle. Then, I build the story toward a positive place. I talk about what this Journey has meant for me: "What I've done is something you can do too. What do you have to give, at this point in your life? What gifts have you experienced through your own Journey?" I ask a lot of rhetorical questions to plant seeds in people's minds. Then I try to end on an inspiring, uplifting note—something that makes them feel like they've just been given the keys to the kingdom.

By the way, if you're reading that, thinking, "Hey—that's exactly what Brenda did with this book,"—you're damn right. If you've read this far, it must be working!

So, consider: What message do *you* want to share with other patients and their families? What wisdom can *you* offer to people, after going through what you have? That message may change, depending on who you choose to share it with. For instance, the advice I share with MS patients is different from a legacy story I want to leave my daughter and granddaughter. Your audience will help shape the story you tell.

What wisdom can you offer, having navigated your own Patient's Journey? What lessons have you learned? What have you overcome? What do you know now that you didn't at the start?

Once you've thought about *what* you want to share—think of *how* you want to share it.

Ways to Share Your Story

In this day and age, there's no shortage of ways to share your story. Here are a few ideas:

- **Keep it simple:** Share it with your family and/or friends, so they have greater insight into what your experience has been.
- **Share it with a community group:** Your spiritual community, your civic organization, your volunteer group, or your local patient support network.
- **Share it more broadly:** Believe it or not, once you share your story a few times, people might start *asking* you to come and share it at other venues. Many organizations are always on the hunt for speakers, and many of those opportunities will be compensated. You may balk at that, or it may feel like an incredibly meaningful and validating opportunity—your call.
- **Use tech platforms:** There are many ways you can use social media, podcasts, websites, blogs, YouTube, and other forums to get your story out there, both in video and written form.

The point is, just take the time to get your experience out of your head and heart, and onto some paper. Then, share it with someone else.

A tip: be smart about when you sit down to do this. If you're in the midst of chemo and radiation, for instance, this is probably not the time to sit down and tackle a writing project. Remember what you've learned about energy conservation! Use your good moments

to lean into this. Opportunities to share will come, and I encourage
you to say yes or no to those, according to the boundaries that make
sense for you.

Why Share?

I remember watching Selma Blair perform on *Dancing with the
Stars*. I tuned in to every episode because Selma Blair is a fellow
MS patient. And every week, Selma went out there and danced her
ass off. She spun, she dipped, she got flipped around in the air. After
each performance, the entire cast—all the celebrities, all the judges,
many people in the audience—were all in tears. Massive boohooing.
Why? Because it was raw and real and so damn inspiring seeing
her achieve something she never thought she could.

When you choose to share your story, that will be the imprint:
you feel like you have been able to overcome and achieve something
you never thought you could. The experience will be profoundly
beneficial for you.

In fact, you will benefit from sharing your story even if it's just with
yourself in the mirror. I used to share my story with myself driving in
the car—I did that hundreds of times. And as I repeated the narrative
of my own Patient's Journey, it's like I was wearing down the path to
walk it, which enabled me to move through the next lap more quickly
and with greater ease. I start with Grief and Anger—"I cried. I felt
incredible sadness. I was like, 'Are you joking?! I've been diagnosed
with some shit that nobody wants.'" Then on into the season of Acceptance, learning to let go of the grief and suffering; learning to build in
Endurance, tend to my relationships, seek out necessary information.
And then Rebuilding: "What do I want to put into my life now? How
do I want things to look with my family, my relationships, friendships,

job, volunteer commitments, and organizations?" By the time I get to the final stage—focusing on Impact—I'm able to look back and say, "Damn! I'm doing pretty good!" And what a happiness boost that is! Even if it's just me in my car.

If and when you do share your story with others, it most certainly will benefit them as well. I've seen it a thousand times. In fact, I have a folder saved on my computer where I have thousands of emails saved, sent by patients who heard one of our Patient Ambassadors speak and had to say thank you. We even pay for a storage facility where I can open old steel filing cabinets and take out cards we were sent twenty years ago. I can look at an analytics report and see countless data points related to a Patient Ambassador story-share, and how it moved the needle for not just the person sharing but also all the people listening.

I've met patient after patient after patient who all said the same thing: "If I can help just one person, it's worth it to share my story. If I can make an imprint on just *one* person's heart, I can die happy." Then, they share—and the flood gates open.

I *know* it to be true because I have seen it, experienced it, watched it, and lived it. Your story has the power to impact.

That's the gift! That's what good looks like. That's one of the biggest ways you get to reclaim peace within yourself. And I don't say this as a Pollyanna—we all know that chronic illness is hell to deal with. But telling your story *makes it easier.* It makes it better, more real, and it helps others.

One of the biggest ways to reclaim peace within yourself is through sharing your story.

There's power in being a role model, and you can absolutely be a role model to yourself. By choosing to do the brave thing and share your story, you're giving the ultimate gift to someone else: the confidence that *they* can go forward, as you have chosen to do. You remind *yourself* that you can keep going. And you might just be a catalyst for someone's choice to go left instead of right—to choose hope instead of despair, or to take the courageous step rather than staying hidden away.

In that folder on my computer, and in many of those heavy file drawers in the storage unit, there are thousands of messages that were sent by the Patient Ambassadors themselves. The sentiment they express is the same: "Thank you for empowering me to connect with others and share my story of hope, grace, and positivity. Not only did I help other people, but without realizing it, I also helped myself. The craziest part of the work I've done to share my story has been that I actually fixed myself."

MESSAGE TO CARE PARTNERS

Enjoy watching your person soar! If and when your loved one starts giving back and inspiring others—that is a huge reason to celebrate for *both* of you. Take some pride and joy in the fact that *you* helped get your loved one to a place where they desire to make an impact. You helped contribute to the well-being of your sick person on the road to healing, both emotionally and physically. If they become a rockstar in this Impact phase—cheer them on, knowing that you played a key role in their success. Supporting your loved one's upward trajectory is a beautiful form for your own impact to take.

If the patient in your life has reached this stage, enjoy the relief that comes with it! Breathe a sigh of relief: "Okay—we *can* go on.

Life is going to be okay. We've got this." You've come a long way in this journey. You've endured a lot, put up with a lot, you've experienced all the same highs and lows they have, but in a different form. For both of you, getting to the Impact stage is like reaching the land of milk and honey after a long and miserable trek through the desert. Celebrate your shared arrival to this happier, healthier place on the Patient's Journey.

But if the patient in your life *doesn't* reach this stage—if their illness has led to cognitive decline, significant and permanent impairment, or even death—your impact as a care partner may look different. I know parents whose daughter was born with terminal congenital deformities. They knew from the day of her birth that she would have a very short life. Their impact was about ensuring that she had as many good days as possible, and that she always felt their love. And that investment on their part, combined with the powerful story they shared with others after their daughter died, was deeply meaningful.

In cases like that, the Impact stage of the Patient's Journey may be primarily yours to make. I know other parents of a young boy who had epilepsy and tragically passed away from a violent seizure. After mourning for a time, they started a hugely successful foundation in his memory to further epilepsy research. Their ability to rise out of significant grief and focus on ways to further their son's legacy through research was a profound form of impact. Another friend of mine is married to a woman with a chronic condition requiring regular care. My friend realized that, when he passed away, his wife wouldn't be able to afford to pay a live-in care provider but also wouldn't qualify for social services reserved for people under the poverty line. He founded an organization that provides benefits and respite care for people who aren't "poor enough" to qualify for social services but still need care at an affordable cost, filling the gap for people like him and his wife.

Here's the point: don't underestimate your own potential for impact—even if your loved one doesn't "get well" in the traditional sense. You may be fortunate enough to cheer on the patient in your life as they inspire others and make an impact. You may need to focus on the smaller but no less profound impact of providing your loved one with the best care possible. Or, you may seek ways to make your own impact in memory of your loved one. Each form of investment is powerful and meaningful.

Finally, never forget the power of stories. Care partners can and should also share their stories. Consider which elements of your care partner story will have the most impact when shared, and use it to encourage other care partners who are earlier in the journey.

YOUR LEGACY

For some patients, especially those with a terminal diagnosis, the focus of your Impact will be your legacy. And rather than dwelling on the sadness of that fact, I want you to think of that as an opportunity. This is a profound gift you can leave to the people you love.

If there are relationships in your life that have caused you pain or consternation, do what you can to set those right. Life is too short for regret to weigh heavily on your heart. You might choose to impact your world for good by cleaning house in that way, and seeking healing in some of those fraught relationships.

Once again, sharing your story can help this process. Make a video of yourself telling your story, dictate it into an app, or write down a message. Taking the time to capture your heartfelt story in those ways can go a long way, not only in healing you but by providing comfort to the people that matter.

Shaping your legacy is not exclusive to people with a terminal condition, either. I think this concept is at the forefront of anyone's mind dealing with a serious diagnosis. Every new MS flare-up I have reminds me that nothing is guaranteed. It doesn't take away my joy or positivity, but in the back of my mind, that eventual reality is there: *Is this my time?* Even though I've lived with MS for over thirty years now, illness is a fluid experience. I know things can change fast. And that makes crafting a legacy even more important.

That's why I continue to write things down and reflect. I continue to bring myself to a place of positivity and hope. In fact, one of the reasons I decided to write this book is because I want my daughter and granddaughter to have a legacy from me. I wanted to provide them with a testimony of my story, along with the principles that I value deeply.

You may share your impact far and wide from a podium, or you may simply impact yourself, in a private letter. You may impact a large audience, or focus your impact exclusively on your family. Your impact may last for years, growing and expanding in its influence, or it may occur within a short window and live on as a legacy after that.

But however your impact is shared, however it penetrates, know this: your Patient's Journey has not been in vain. Your story matters. Your experience has the power to change lives.

Your story matters. Your experience has the power to change lives.

STANDING OVATION

In early 2019, I got a phone call. "Hello, Brenda Snow?" the voice on the other line inquired. "This is Anna. I'm the publisher of PM360." PM360 is one of the top trade publications for biopharma marketers. "Yes?" I replied. "How can I help you?"

She said, "We've watched your career over the years, and we would like to honor you with the Trailblazer Lifetime Achievement Award this year. Would you accept it?"

Instantly, I became choked up. The people that had won that award before were the movers and shakers in our industry. Although I was a founder and CEO, I still thought of myself as an MS patient. Typically, they weren't handing out these awards to patients. "You want to give *me* a Lifetime Achievement Award?" I asked, almost in disbelief.

Anna laughed on the other end. "You and your team have turned an industry on its head," she said. "We think the Trailblazer label fits you to a tee."

I vividly remember the day of the ceremony. It was an evening event, and I wanted to look fabulous. I had chosen a long black gown to wear—black, because it was slimming. (It's only been in the past two years that I've finally, *finally* lost all that extra weight I put on from the steroids and all those tacos.) I wanted to wear a great pair of shoes to go with the dress, but I also knew that I was going to have to climb up stairs, walk across a stage, stand at a podium, and give a keynote address—and, hello, MS patient. So, I opted to wear a lovely pair of shoes with a wide toe base and one-inch heels. In my MS life, I embrace comfortable shoes. For sparkle and glamour, I wore a massive necklace covered in fake diamonds.

Before the ceremony, I gathered the team that had traveled there with me and passed out champagne. "I want everyone here to know that I consider this award a shared success. I hope you pass that message on to your teams: I did *not* do this alone. I did it with the help of every single one of you here with me, and everyone else on your teams." We clinked our champagne flutes, and I had a few sips—but not too much. I didn't want to fall down walking up to the podium!

When the moment finally arrived and I was on the stage, Corbin presented me with the award. There's a picture of us in that moment, and we both have the biggest, cheesiest grins on our faces. I could never have done it without him!

I talked about what it meant to be recognized as someone who disrupted an industry. I made some jokes. But the most important message I shared was about what it means to be a patient. "This is a universal fact of life," I said. "We're all going to be touched by disease and illness at some point. So, it is vital that we stay connected with the people we're doing this work for." I looked out at the faces in the audience—people working at the highest levels of biotech and pharma, people dressed to the nines, and people who—for the next few minutes—*had* to listen to whatever I wanted to say.

"I want to ask every person in this room to please remember that we are here in the service of patients. If you're in this room, you've likely had a wonderful career. You've made a lot of money; you've lived the life you wanted to. But lest we forget, please stay connected to the patients you serve. You are developing novel therapeutics to help change the course of some of the diseases. The minute you stop thinking about your patients as *people*, and instead, think of them as a *tactic,* you will fail. Remember *the people* who are behind your success."

When I finished my speech, the applause started—and then people stood on their feet.

It had been twenty-six years since I'd wondered if I was going to orphan my daughter; twenty-five since being in that inpatient rehab ward; and eighteen since getting kicked out of a San Francisco boardroom by men who dismissed patient stories as a "cute" idea. And that standing ovation felt pretty fucking good. It was the ultimate validation after years of struggle and hard work: this amazing acknowledgment by a group of my peers, in the company of my incredible business partner and my great colleagues.

I was never alone. The impact that I've been privileged to make was done in the company of an incredible team. And the Journey I have navigated as a patient was done in the company of dear family, friends, and a wide array of fabulous healthcare professionals.

You are not alone.

As you walk this Journey—or limp, or roll, or recline—remember that you are in the company of other courageous souls who have gone before you and journey beside you. Each one of us has *powerful* potential to impact this world for good—even though, and especially because, we are patients.

STAGE 10 OF THE PATIENT'S JOURNEY: IMPACT

- *Common emotions: a desire to give back, make a difference, shape your legacy; inspiration to venture out in ways you haven't before with the new lessons you've learned.*

- *Common pitfalls: assuming you don't have much to offer or that your story doesn't matter; putting off shaping your story, contribution, or legacy.*

- *Your best next step: Carve out time to intentionally reflect on your story and consider how you might want to contribute to others with the new gifts you've gathered during this Journey. Then, take a step toward making that Impact. The world will be better for it!*

Conclusion

"Being challenged in life is inevitable. Being defeated is optional."

— Roger Crawford

What will your story be? Even now, you're in the midst of forming it as you navigate your own Patient's Journey. In the weeks, months, and years to come, your story will take shape: the ways you overcame your hardest moments, the breakthroughs you experienced in your relationships, the new purpose and meaning you discovered; the strategies you discovered to manage your disease, and the reinvention and impact you realized were yours to make.

What will your story be?

I can think of so many patients who have walked this road, shared their stories, and impacted the world for good. It has been a sacred gift in my life that so many of those patients opened their hearts to me—essentially a stranger when I initially met them—and

339

shared their biggest, darkest moments, their fears, their insecurities about where they were when they struggled with their diagnoses, and their tentative hopes. Maybe it's my internal optimism, but I have never met a single patient where, after we spoke, I walked away thinking, *Yeah, they can't do it*, or *They don't get it. They're going to end up staying like this.*

They *did* do it. They *did* get it. They moved *through* their Patient's Journey and chose hope and wholeness along the way.

I think of Christy—a dynamic, incredible woman who found early success as a high-powered corporate lawyer. Like me, Christy began to experience symptoms of MS in her early thirties. The cognitive issues that came with it started to compromise her abilities as a lawyer, and she struggled to keep up with the challenges of law. She was marginalized by her colleagues and eventually ousted from her firm. She lost the career that had been the center of her life, and because she had put off dating for the sake of her career, she didn't have a partner to help her navigate her diagnosis. As was the case in my story, that diagnosis was hell to come by. More than one doctor told Christy that she was simply hysterical.

But Christy had enough gumption to persist, and a few years into her diagnosis, she started the right treatments and put the right strategies in place. She even fell in love—after being told that no one would want her now that she was sick. She's had a decades-long lovely marriage and went on to become a federally appointed judge. Then, after her tenure there, she returned to practicing law. Christy has told me that she's so much happier with the life she's arrived at than she would have been with a life where she was spending eighty hours a week grinding it out as a corporate lawyer. She's made her way to a life of wholeness and joy.

I think about Henrietta,* a wonderful woman who was struggling to accept herself on many levels. Henrietta was diagnosed with schizophrenia, which is already a stigmatizing disease. But on top of that, she was a gay woman living in a rural, southern town and doing her best to hide her condition and her sexuality from her community. When I met her, she had no self-worth, and she was convinced she had nothing to offer people. Her self-esteem was so low, she didn't believe her perspective mattered. She didn't think her story would resonate or make an impact on anyone. I told her, "You have to *not* give up on yourself." Henrietta didn't see what I could: her amazing, incredible presence.

Henrietta had tried so hard to "heal" parts of her that didn't need healing—they just needed to be accepted. One of my fondest memories is the time I got to see Henrietta shine in an amazing performance at a karaoke bar. She finally owned who she was *and* her disease, and she is a beacon to so many people dealing with social stigmas because of things they can't change. She showed such courage as she stepped out of hiding and overcame her fears to be honest about who she was.

I think of Joe,† a person of color with sickle cell anemia. Because of systematic marginalization around both his race and diagnosis, he was underserved by the medical community and felt like he didn't have a voice to advocate for himself. But eventually, Joe practiced crafting his story and claiming a platform. He was able to find a successful treatment plan after developing the courage to push back on the system and share his story broadly. Now, this

---

* Name changed to protect privacy.

† Name changed to protect privacy.

incredible man is a pillar of his community and a respected voice to healthcare professionals.

The list goes on and on. I think of marriages that *didn't* blow up, partners who stayed together because they worked as a team and tried to navigate the Patient's Journey side by side, which brought them closer, rather than driving them apart. Many of these marriages were initially very troubled by the stress brought on by disease, but by utilizing a lot of the tips and strategies we've talked about in this book, they ended up telling me this experience of dealing with disease together was the best thing that could have happened to their relationship. It strengthened their communication and ability to be vulnerable with each other, which brought them to a place of greater emotional depth and authenticity. I've seen countless couples go on to have a deeper, fabulous marriage after a diagnosis.

From hell to wholeness: their story. *Your* story.

From hell to wholeness: their story. Your story.

Where are you on the Patient's Journey? We've talked about each stage:

- **Pre-Diagnosis,** a time characterized by fear, confusion, and sometimes denial. The best thing you can do for yourself in this stage is confront what's going on in your body and seek out answers.
- **Diagnosis,** a stage of strange bedfellows, when fear and relief intertwine. This is also a time that feels vaguely surreal, involves a deluge of information, and may

include especially acute symptoms. Because a diagnosis can create an "identity earthquake," it's especially important during this time to shore up your connection to others and, especially, to yourself.

• **Grief** comes next, with all its different shades: grief surrounding relief, comprehension, future fears, empathy, reentry, and loss. Although you may not feel optimistic in this stage, it's crucial to choose a hopeful outlook, so that you can make choices for yourself that lead you toward greater healing.

• **Anger** follows hard after Grief, or the two may be closely layered. It's easy to get consumed by anger and stuck there, but you're better off harnessing the energy from anger to pull you toward productive outcomes. Think of your disease as a competition you need to win and shape an inner narrative that helps you move forward beyond the victim mindset.

• **Acceptance** takes you across a threshold to a place that feels more calm, productive, and empowered. By holding the burdens of disease in balance with the gifts, you open yourself up to healing and remember what it is to love yourself.

• **Endurance** characterizes the lengthy season that follows, when you learn to incorporate rhythms of personal self-care and implement processes that help set you up for a sustainable lifestyle. This is also a time to proactively care for the people supporting you.

• **Optimize Your Relationships** puts the spotlight on your emotional care team. We talked about optimizing your healthy relationships and giving yourself permission to get certain unhelpful people off your team. Patients, care partners, family members, and friends will all evolve as you move through the Patient's Journey—both individuals, and the relationships between individuals will be affected. Those evolutions can be a really good thing.

- **Optimize Your Care** is when you begin to aggressively self-advocate—or deputize your care partner to aggressively advocate for you—so you get the information you need. We talked about getting the right healthcare team in place, and I pointed you toward other avenues where you might seek out information and support. This is a stage where you want to put energy and focus into defining and redefining your healthcare plan.

- **Rebuilding** is a time of renewal, reinvention, and fun. You get to take back happy! As you architect normalcy back into your life, you also want to plan for fun, joy-filled times. This stage is also characterized by decisions to redirect your path toward areas of investment that you find truly meaningful.

- **Impact** signals the culmination of your Patient's Journey, when you embrace the avenues where you are uniquely qualified to make a difference in the world because of your diagnosis. Your impact may be personal and occur mainly within your family, or you may choose to pursue broader platforms of impact. However you choose to shape your contribution, make sharing your story a part of it.

If there's one thing you take away from this book, I hope it's that you now know you have the power to be more than your symptoms. You are *more* than your illness. You can overcome these challenges—which at times, I know, seem insurmountable. Yet, the power we all have within ourselves is amazing.

You are *more* than your illness. You can overcome these challenges!

Sometimes I think the experience of getting a chronic or even terminal illness gives us license to flip on the switch that lets all our superpowers shine out. We are so much more than these illnesses! I am more than MS. You are more than Crohn's disease or cancer or HIV or epilepsy or long Covid.

You *can* overcome it, but you've got to move through the hell. You'll need to work on Acceptance—and that's probably the hardest mountain to climb. You need to make peace with your disease, and then you'll need to endure the ups and downs, putting time and energy into architecting a new life for yourself.

The goal you're aiming toward is wholeness, which I define as ultimate happiness. When I look back at my own Journey, I realize that I've never been happier. Even as a kid, I don't know that I envisioned a life that could be this happy. And I think much of that joy has come from my Patient's Journey and my experience with MS. Through navigating these things, I've been able to focus on what really matters in life and be deliberate about crafting my experiences toward wholeness. As I've shared in this book, I used to get consumed by some of the stupidest things—staying late at work to impress the boss, having a perfectly clean house, or worrying about what my neighbors thought of me. I put time and energy into some of these culturally conventional things that distracted me from what was most important.

My chronic disease pried all that away from me, forcing me to let go of the stupid stuff that doesn't matter. It prompted me to prioritize the things that have brought joy into my life, opening my eyes to see greater beauty and feel tremendous gratitude. I've gone beyond work/life balance—I've learned how to spend my gifts and time in a way that cultivates deeper meaning for myself, my family, and my partner. That's the gift of wholeness that multiple sclerosis has brought me.

That's what I want for you!

So, I'm passing you the baton. It's time to put your plan together. Take in these recommendations, find out what they mean to you, and then put your plan into action.

It's important for you to understand that the wholeness you *can* arrive at through the Patient's Journey is not guaranteed. There's no magic wand to take you from bitter, angry victimhood to joyful wholeness. You do need to actually do the work. You can read this book and say, "This is all great!" but if you don't implement the strategies I've given you, progress will be slow or stagnate altogether.

The wholeness you *can* arrive at through the Patient's Journey is not guaranteed. There's no magic wand to take you from bitter, angry victimhood to joyful wholeness. You need to actually do the work.

So, consider: Given where you're at on the Patient's Journey, what strategies are immediately applicable? What are specific steps you can take to put those into practice and actually move yourself forward on this Journey? Identify those. Write them down. Share them with someone. Put this into action! You may choose just one thing to start doing right away. If that's the case, good. Bravo! If you try ten strategies, terrific. But the point is don't stop and give up when you have a shit day. We *all* have shit days and it's okay to just let one of those be. Then, the next day, start again. Keep trying.

It's taken me decades to truly hone my own Patient's Journey. I hadn't mastered it in my first two years. Some of the strategies that I describe in Endurance, Optimize Your Relationships, and Optimize Your Care took years to fine tune, and I'm constantly retooling. There are still days when I have to work through Acceptance of new symptoms or elements of how my disease manifests. So, give yourself time and grace—but don't give up. Don't ever give up. Keep trying.

Give yourself time and grace as you put in the work to move forward on this Journey—but don't give up. Don't ever give up. Keep trying.

You may not feel like you can do this—but *I know you can.* When you are feeling down and overwhelmed, take this advice from a seasoned patient. Even when you don't believe in yourself, I believe in you. And I want you to believe me, because I KNOW you can do this. I've known many patients who thought the exact same thing as you, who had days when they believed they couldn't do it. And yet, I've seen those people get to the other side.

Your darkest moments, your saddest times, your rudderless feelings—those will get better. You will make peace with those emotions. The hard times will come and go on your Patient's Journey, but you will start to own them and overcome them. You will start to grow. If you remember half the nuggets in this book, you will have a life of richness and beauty.

Choose hope. Chase wholeness. Recognize the good life that is ahead of you—and *live*!

Acknowledgments

Undertaking a project like this was a bit overwhelming at times, filled with fear, self-doubt, anticipation, and ultimately joy as it has come to fruition. This book is a result of many teachers and inspiring people who supported me and I'd like to thank and acknowledge a few.

First: my amazing daughter, Stephanie, who has been my biggest inspiration to get and stay "well." You always believed in me, even when I didn't. Your beautiful, sensitive spirit and love for me was a constant I always felt, especially during tough times on my journey with MS. You are my best friend and I am so thankful I am your mommy. You make me want to be better every day. I love you.

My husband, Oliver, whose unwavering support in all aspects of my life is unparalleled. You are a huge source of strength for me and I'd be at a loss without you. I'm eternally grateful for your intellect and keen editing eye, countless hours listening to me talk about this fucking book, and believing I could even when I didn't. You are a wonderful husband and I love you with my whole heart. Now let's travel!

My parents, Ron and Sharon Snow, whose spectacular DNA combo produced the winning ticket with me! Seriously, your life lessons, humor, tenacity, hard work, and the way you conduct your lives has been the biggest example and role model of what "good" looks like for me and my lovely sister, Debbie. Thank you Mom and Dad for loving me and always being a safe place.

My aunt, Melinda Snow, who has been my partner in crime for the last fifty-five years. You've seen it all, "wiped it all," picked up the pieces, saved my life (twice!), and been a constant source of friendship and stability for me and Steph. Now we've just got to get through old age!

My business partner and bestie, Corbin Wood. I feel honored to have learned from you, laughed with you, shared an office with you, enjoyed wildly inappropriate conversations with you, and built our great company together. The ride of a lifetime. There's nobody else I'd rather have in my corner than you. Simply put, the best.

My Snow Team, past and present. I consider myself very lucky to have been surrounded by brilliant, dedicated individuals who sacrificed their time and energy to build a great company and, more importantly, help so many people. I'm grateful to you for believing in me as your leader, a job I take very seriously. You are tremendous and my heart is full thinking of you all. I'd like to especially recognize Mike Simone and Nadine McGown who have been instrumental in building Snow while ensuring we always stayed close to our ethics, mission, and culture of putting patients first. The best friends a girl could ask for, thank you.

Our clients, past and present. Without your belief in our abilities and taking a risk to support patients and their families in a novel and new way, none of this would have happened. I am filled with gratitude for each and every one of you.

To Greta the Great, the best partner when one decides to undertake the ridiculous idea of writing a book. Your patience, smile, and brilliance pulled us through. Thanks for helping me make this a reality!

Avery, my adorable granddaughter. May this book be an inspiration to you as you grow up knowing that you come from strong women who believe in themselves and, with effort, have the ability to make the world a better place (swear words and all)! You are the biggest joy in my life and I look forward to watching you craft your own story, darling girl.

Finally, the heroes: to all of the Patient Ambassadors and their families that touched my life in unfathomable ways. Your lives are deep with meaning and demonstrate the best of the human spirit. I carry your stories with me, treasure the time I've spent with you, and feel humbled that you let strangers into your Journeys so all of us together could make a very big impact: sharing how to live with meaning and purpose in spite of chronic illness. As I reflect on my life, it is each of you who have truly made my hardest days bearable and whose strength I call upon when needed. I'm in awe of your courage. Thank you for sharing your beautiful souls with me.

Be well on your Patient Journey and know you are not alone. It will all be okay. Promise!

Love, Brenda

About the Author

B renda Snow has pioneered patient engagement for the life science industry with her agency, Snow Companies, which she leads as the founder and CEO. Grown out of Brenda's own experience as a patient with multiple sclerosis, Snow Companies, now part of Omnicom Health Group, employs more than 400 staff worldwide.

Under Brenda's leadership, Snow Companies has won over 200 awards, including PM360's Trailblazer Agency of the Year, *Inc.* magazine's Fastest Growing Private Companies, and AMCP's MarCom Award. PharmaVoice has repeatedly listed Brenda among the life science industry's most inspiring people, and numerous NGOs worldwide recognize her for the achievements she has won on behalf of the patient community.

Brenda is passionately involved in local and global humanitarian and artistic causes. She has served on various boards and mentored many individuals to help them escape dead ends and unlock their true potential.